Long Term Care
YOUR ROLE IN QUALITY & RESIDENT MEALTIME EXPERIENCE WORKBOOK

A Regulatory Compliance Guide for Nursing Home Administrators, Directors of Nursing, Nurse Managers, Dietitians, Food Service Directors/Managers, Certified Nurse Aides/Nursing Assistants, Food Service Aides, and for others of the Nursing Home Community

NORA WELLINGTON

authorHOUSE

AuthorHouse™
1663 Liberty Drive
Bloomington, IN 47403
www.authorhouse.com
Phone: 833-262-8899

Published by AuthorHouse 12/01/2023

ISBN: 979-8-8230-1718-3 (sc)
ISBN: 979-8-8230-1717-6 (e)

Library of Congress Control Number: 2023922276

Print information available on the last page.

Contents

PART 6

Acknowledgments

I want to thank my family for your love, for your continued support, for making our family enjoy that closeness that we are blessed with, and for helping me stay motivated and feel so good at what I do. I am especially grateful to my two sons, as you continue to be my sounding board, bouncing ideas off of you as I advance professionally and take on new projects. I am very grateful for you all.

To the staffs and colleagues of the long term care facilities that gave me the opportunity to serve them, I am grateful that you made me a better administrator. Also I thank the CEO's, Partners, Regional Directors of the National and Regional Long Term Care Organizations that took a chance on me, when I became a long term care management consultant. I say thank you as this gave me opportunity to continue developing my passion for long term care, my leadership skills, introduction to different systems, best practices and Continuous Quality Improvements in each environment.

To members of my Editorial Board: my colleagues and friends: Andrea Brown, Olabisi Daramy, Lutricia Quarles and Sheila Singletary, I say a very Big Thank You for the developmental editing you provided to this book. You took your valuable time out of your usually busy schedule, to review and edit my work. You provided me with valuable and beneficial suggestions and recommendations. For that I am truly grateful. Your combined experience as long term care professionals in leadership positions proved beneficial to me, as I did incorporated your suggestions and recommendations into the book. You are also my cheerleaders, cheering me on with my work, and I love that. To Gloria Allen, an author as well, thanks for helping me with my final editing. I appreciate your time, your commitment and your diligence.

Thank you Cathy Fyock, Business Book Strategist, and Coach for your invaluable help in also providing editing and input on whether the structure I selected for the book made sense. I appreciate your feedback and guidance in helping me make the book more readable. I appreciate your support.

Finally I am grateful for the blessings which have enabled me to be of service to the residents and staffs of our long term care community.

Dear Reader: nursing home administrator, director of nursing, dietitian, food service director, nurse manager, nurse aides/nursing assistant, food service aides, LTC community

Thank you very much for your interest in this workbook. I am happy that you have decided to see what this workbook offers. Topic covered here are about Quality, the regulations F-tags, resident mealtime, and case studies in skilled nursing facilities (SNFs) and other long term care facilities. If you are an employee in long term facilities, I am doubly grateful that you are reading this book.

I am a thirty plus (30+) years nursing home administrator. I continue to wonder that as Much as the Centers for Medicare & Medicaid Services (CMS) continues to update the regulations and other quality initiatives, there continues to be concerns about quality in nursing homes. Through the years in my career, I developed a passion for resident/ patient care, for regulatory compliance and for quality. As a former business office manager with an MBA, I surprised myself when I became so passionate about resident care. Early in my career, I was fortunate to be hired to help a hospital open a brand new Subacute/Skilled Nursing Unit for a hospital; and this is how I started to develop my passion. The nurses at this hospital-based SNF facility called me an "honorary nurse". It was such an honor.

Now to the reason why I decided to write this workbook – we all know that the long term care regulations are so voluminous, and trying to take all that information in gets overwhelming and stressful sometimes. My goal in writing this workbook - "Long Term Care Your Role In Quality and Resident Mealtime Experience" is to help minimize some of that feeling of stress, by breaking up the F-tags into focus sections of care areas, departments and disciplines. You can go to your section in the workbook, see your F-tags that you need to focus on as you do your job, embrace those F-tags, internalize those F-tags and do your work to provide the quality of care and services, quality of life and resident safety for your residents. I know your work is demanding at all levels. I have been there as administrator, and now as a long term care management consultant, I still help facilities.

The departments/positions that are covered in this workbook with their F-tags focus are Administrators, Directors of Nursing, Dietitians, Food Service Directors/Managers, Nurse Managers and Certified Nurse Aides/Nursing Assistants, Food Service Aides, and QAPI Director/Coordinator. I hope you will find this workbook very user friendly and helpful.

You can find me at www.norawellingtonbooks.com. And I will have some free downloads on monitoring audit tools and other items.

Thanks again,

Sincerely,
Nora Wellington, MBA, LNHA, Author

Introduction

With always the concern for quality in nursing homes, how are we going to break that tide? The good news is that some of the facilities have broken that tide; they are providing quality of care and services for their residents and keeping the focus on continuous performance improvement. Others however are lagging behind, with some of these facilities having an Overall Quality Rating of "One Star – Much Below Average" out of Five Star in the Medicare Nursing Home Compare system. As some of the facilities continue to fall short on standards, regulatory compliance, and expectations, complaints continue to grow and take root.

The Office of the Inspector General (OIG) for the Department of Health and Human Services conducts oversight and evaluates the Centers for Medicare & Medicaid Services' performance over the nations' nursing homes. OIG provides reports for Congress showing how well or not the nation's nursing homes are performing. As quality has been and continues to be an ongoing issue and concern for some residents, families, advocates, stakeholders and for some of the nursing homes themselves, CMS through the years have developed quality initiatives. In 1987 the first major overhaul and enhancement of the Federal Long Term Care Regulations, was the Omnibus Budget Reconciliation Act known, as OBRA 1987.

As staffing is part of the data collected towards this system, and because some facilities struggle in the area of staffing, the level of staffing in the facilities has also become an issue related to the quality of care and services. Staffing is also a component of the Five-Star Quality Rating System. So now in addition to the number of staff or the level of staff in the facilities, CMS had placed focus on the competences of the staff, and revised parts of the reformed regulations to include staff competencies in addition to the number of licensed staff and turnover of leadership staff in the facility.

Workbook Goals and Objectives

This workbook is designed:

- To help the administrator establish and maintain a culture in your facility where staffs embrace the importance of being knowledgeable of the long term care regulations F-tags,
- To help make it a little easy for department heads and their staffs to navigate the regulations and keep the focus on the specific F-tags that pertain to their departments and their areas of responsibility in order to provide quality for the residents
- To help staff become more familiar with their specific regulations and maintain regulatory compliance in their specific areas for resident mealtime
- To help staffs provide quality of care and services, quality of life that the residents deserve
- To help the facility focus on, and develop and maintain a robust quality assurance and performance improvement program
- To help the administrator and departments be survey ready at all times, thereby having good certification surveys results and increased quality star rating
- To help staff improve on providing a pleasant mealtime experience

How to Use This Book – Formatted for Ease of Use by Positions, Disciplines, and Departments

The Positions, Disciplines and Departments Covered in this Workbook

- Administrators – Self-reflection Questions, Specific F-tags regulations, Practical Tips, Case Study
- Directors of Nursing – Self-Reflection Questions, Specific F-tags regulations, Practical Tips, Case Study
- Dietitians Discipline – Self-Reflection Questions, Specific F-tags regulations, Practical Tips, Case Study
- Directors/Managers of Food Service – Self-Reflection Questions, Specific F-tags regulations, Practical Tips, Case Study
- Nurse Managers and Certified Nurse Aides/Nursing Assistants – Self-Reflection Questions for Nurse Managers, Specific F-tags regulations, Practical Tips,
- Quality Assurance and Performance Improvement (QAPI) Directors/ Coordinators – Specific F-tags regulations for QAPI for all departments

For the F-Tags in the Workbook

The specific F-tags covered and addressed in the workbook, carry the language of the regulations in the State Operations Manual Appendix PP for Guidance to Surveyors for Long Term Care Facilities. The INTENT and also the DEFINITIONS also carry the language of the regulations.

For some of the guidance referenced in the workbook, I gave you an abridged form of the guidance for the F-tags with notation for you to refer to the State Operations Manual Appendix PP for Guidance to Surveyors for Long Term Care Facilities, for the full content of the guidance.

Remarks - I have added comments and remarks to highlight some areas of focus

Areas of F-tags Focus Covered in this book

- Residents Quality of Life
- Residents Quality of Care and Services
- Resident Safety
- Resident Rights
- Resident Mealtimes
- Food and Nutrition Services
- Administrators F-tags & role and responsibilities
- Directors of Nursing F-tags and role and responsibilities
- Dietitian F-tags and role and responsibilities
- Food Service Directors/Managers F-tags and role and responsibilities
- Quality Assurance and Performance Improvement (QAPI)

Addressing the Self-Reflective Questions for Department Heads

These questions are for self-assessment and reflection as to where you believe you are in your skill set and in your awareness of the regulations. You can work on these questions by yourselves, or if you want a trusted colleague to give you objective feedback you can invite them to have a discussion with you on these questions.

Handling Tips for Department Heads

These are also areas that you can assess if you are currently performing some of these tips in your daily, weekly or monthly routines. See if these tips are helpful to you. Of course all facilities are different in their corporate structure, and some of the tips may or may not apply to you. These are decision you have to make personally. These are tips, they are not mandates from the author, you will make the decision.

Case Studies and Exercises for Department Heads

Disclaimers for the case studies:

DISCLAIMER: The workbook case studies are fictional –fictional names of skilled nursing facilities and/or nursing homes, fictional situations and fictional stories. The names, characters and incidents portrayed in the case studies are fictional, and no identification with persons (living or dead) and with places or with products should be assumed or inferred.

You can work independently or with colleagues to review the case studies and work on the questions on the "Exercise To Do" at the end of each case studies. If there are additional points you wish to include in the exercise you most certainly can.

PART

I

Chapter 1

RESIDENT MEALTIME DINING EXPERIENCE

Pleasant Meal Time

Residents' mealtime in nursing homes requires the interdepartmental and interdisciplinary approach to attain and maintain a successful mealtime experience for the residents. As stated, the licensed nursing home administrators, directors of nursing, dietitians, food service directors/manager, nurse managers, certified nursing assistants/nurse aides, and food service aides, all have direct and indirect roles and responsibilities to ensure that the goal of pleasant mealtime experience becomes a daily positive outcome for the residents. The expectations established by CMS for residents to receive quality of life as part of their mealtime experience is one of the fundamental components for the Conditions of Participation for the Medicare and Medicaid Program that facilities must attain and maintain.

As administrators, you bear an awesome responsibility to make certain that, your staffs meet the nutritional needs of the residents, as well as the need for residents to have a pleasant mealtime experience. Resident-centered care, individualized care, taking consideration residents' choices and preferences have been incorporated into developing and maintaining quality of care for residents. It is written into the regulation for administrators that residents under your care in your facility attain and maintain their highest practicable physical, mental, and psychosocial well-being. Pleasant resident mealtime and proper nutritional status contribute to the residents attaining and maintaining their physical, mental, and psychosocial well-being.

It is essential that the residents in the nursing homes have the right diet order, the right food on the menu, eating their meals at the right time, and in the right setting they choose. The approach and practice of resident-centered care, individualized care, with residents exercising their preferences in collaboration with the dietitian assessment to determine the appropriate nutritional status, contribute to pleasant resident meal time experience, and quality of life. The physical environment and ambience in the residents dining rooms and the nurse aides' service during meals also contribute positively or negatively depending what your dining room looks like. Does the dining room have a homelike appearance or institutional look? The clinical care and the physical appearance are just as important.

Our next chapter addresses the general topic of Quality in nursing homes.

Chapter 2

QUALITY

Quality of Care & Services in Nursing Homes

The Federal Long Term Care Regulations promulgated by the Centers for Medicare & Medicaid Services (CMS) address the fundamentals of quality of care and services, quality of life, and resident safety in nursing homes. All stakeholders in the nursing home and long term care community know that quality has been and continues to be a focus and desire for the federal government, for the state governments, for families and resident representatives, for the residents, for advocates and for the nursing home staff themselves. Quality issues and concerns continue to be an ongoing concern. Below are some of the initiatives and steps that have been taken to help resolve this problem of quality in nursing homes.

In 1987 the federal government issued what they called a landmark regulation to establish minimum standards for the quality of care and services, and the quality of life that nursing homes certified as Medicare & Medicaid facilities must provide for residents in their care. The regulations were titled The Omnibus Budget Reconciliation Act of 1987, OBRA for short. The regulations required that the nursing homes must provide services for their residents so each resident can "attain and maintain his/her highest practicable physical, mental, and psychosocial well-being." In September 1992, September 1995, and October 2016 the scope of Federal regulations was enhance to include the provision for skilled nursing facilities and nursing facilities to qualify by maintaining the standards for participation in the Medicare & Medicaid programs.

In spite of this and other initiatives quality continued to be a persistent issue and problem for the nursing homes. Complaints about quality from stakeholders and advocates in the nursing home community were persistent. The Office of Inspector General (OIG) has an oversight function for the Department of Health and Human

Services (HHS) to evaluate the performance of nursing homes, and provide reports for Congress. State Survey Agencies and the Federal surveyors conduct annual certification surveys determining the performance of the nursing homes through their survey results/deficiency reports. Analysis of the top ten (10) deficiencies cited for the nursing homes usually include quality of care, quality of life, food procurement and food service, care planning, and infection control. Based on these analyses the issue of quality continues to be a problem. Of course not all facilities have problems with quality of course, but the prevalence of those facilities with problems with quality persist to a certain degree.

Quality Initiatives

Advancing Excellence – was launched in 2006 for nursing homes to help address the quality problem by setting a goal of improving quality in nursing homes. This initiative which was voluntary required nursing homes to sign up to participate with the goal of improving quality of care and services and quality of life for their residents. Nursing homes did sign up to participate. and they committed to focus on three (3) of the eight (8) measurable goals. The facilities benefited from the program.

National Nursing Home Quality Improvement (NNHQI)

In 2016 the Advancing Excellence Collaborative turned over its quality initiative (Advancing Excellence) over to CMS. CMS re-named the quality initiative the National Nursing Home Quality Improvement (NNHQI) Campaign. CMS focus with NNHAQI was to enable continuous quality improvements in nursing homes and provide free evidence based resources to help facilities achieve this goal. Some of the focus included empowering leadership and staffs of the nursing home community, involving the consumers and bringing to light the culture of continuous quality improvement. Also the Long Term Care Ombudsman Programs in all states became involved in the NNHQI campaign.

Office of Inspector General (OIG) Oversight

The Office of Inspector General (OIG) has as a focus preventing fraud, waste and abuse; and improving the efficiency of the Medicare, Medicaid program through CMS and the other DHS programs. OIG has done decades of evaluations of CMS inspections of nursing homes. Below are some of the evaluations and inspections that OIG has reported upon and their findings.

January 2023 – OIG reported on the level of Infection Rates that a thousand plus nursing homes reached an unacceptable rate in the first year of COVID-19 Pandemic.

November 2022, OIG reported on Psychotropic drug use in nursing homes

January 2022 OIG address some states poor performance in conducting nursing home surveys

June 2021 OIG reported on the devastating impact of the COVID-19 on Medicare beneficiaries

September 2020 OIG reported that states continued to fall short in following up on complaints from residents and families in nursing homes.

As stated OIG has been investigating and evaluating nursing homes and providing reports to the Congress of the United States

Five-Star Quality Rating System

The Five-Star-Quality Rating system was designed in 2008 to help residents, families, and consumers understand the assessment and distinction of nursing homes based on their quality. The system which is part of the Medicare.gov website list nursing homes by state and location and with the designation of the overall quality stars (from five stars the highest rating to one star the lowest rating). In addition to the overall rating, the system also gives rating for Health Care Surveys (both standard and complaints surveys), for Quality Measures, and for Staffing. The Five Star Quality Rating System helps families and patient representatives and others who need nursing home placement for their loved ones make choices about nursing homes.

There have been improvements and enhancement in the Five Star Quality system.

- In 2015 CMS made changes to the system that had effect on the Staffing and Quality Measures..
- In 2016 CMs added new Quality Measures to the system.
- In 2018 CMS changed the reporting of staffing information to the utilization of the Payroll-Based Journal for reporting of staffing in nursing homes.

- In 2019 CMS separated the rating for short and long stay residents Quality Measures.
- In 2020 CMS made accommodation for the disruption of the COVID-19 Public Health Emergency.
- In 2023 CMS has made adjustment to staffing by incorporating staffing turnover rate for administrators, and weekend staffing for Registered Nurses.

2016 Comprehensive Revision of the Federal Long Term Care Regulations

Over twenty or thirty plus years it has been determined that residents admitted to nursing homes now require more medical needs and interventions as well as clinically complex needs. Research conducted through the years also revealed the need for providers and their staffs and others in the nursing home community, to have the awareness for residents clinical needs, for the residents' health outcomes, residents' choices and preferences, and more importantly quality assurance and performance improvement.

October 2016 CMS issued a final rule in the federal register for more comprehensive reform of the federal long term care regulations. The final rule titled: Medicare and Medicaid Programs: Reform of Requirements for Long Term-Care Facilities. The revised/reformed regulations confirmed and stressed some of the existing regulations; it also introduced some new requirements for the long term care facilities such as – comprehensive person-centered care planning to compliance and ethics. This Medicare and Medicaid Programs: Reform of Requirements for Long Term Care Facilities. The numbering for the F-tags were also changed and the implementation for the revised regulations were structured into three (3) phases.

- Phase 1 – implementation to be accomplished by facilities by November 28, 2016
- Phase 2 – implementation to be accomplished by facilities by November 28, 2017
- Phase 3 – implementation to be accomplished by facilities by November 28 2019

What was added as Phase 2, regarding quality concerns for nursing homes, is the requirement that when surveyors go to the facilities for surveys, the facilities must provide to surveyors their QAPI Plan, and this became effective after November 28, 2017. Also regarding quality, the revised requirement for participation included facilities to have an Infection Preventionist either on staff or on a consultant basis for each facility, and the Infection Preventionist should participate and be a member of the Quality Assessment and Assurance (QAA) or QAPI committee. This needed to be accomplished by Phase 3, November 28, 2019.

As you can see quality and performance improvement continues to be an ongoing process for the nursing homes. Fortunately there are facilities that are doing very well, with them obtaining 5-Star in their overall quality star rating in the Five Star system, and others which continues to struggle in this area of quality. Quality of care and services, quality of life, and resident safety are the foundation and fundamentals of what facilities do, and it is important that residents receive the care and services they need and deserve.

PART

2

Chapter 3

LISTING OF THE F-TAGS ASSIGNED BY DEPARTMENTS

The specific F-tags I have attributed and delineated for each Discipline and/or Departments are listed below by department. Some of these F-tags are repeated in more than one area of responsibility, due to the importance and relevance in the area of focus.

Below are the F-Tags attributed to the departments and disciplines for focus on Quality and "Resident Mealtime Experience" Please note that I listed the F-Tags by importance and not necessarily in numerical sequence order.

F-tags for the Administrators

F835 - Administration - Administration

F550 – Resident Rights/Exercise Rights – Resident Rights

F584 – Resident Rights – Safe/Clean/Comfortable/Homelike Environment – Resident Rights

F920 – Requirements for Dining and Activity Rooms – Physical Environment

F675 – Quality of Life - Quality

F813 – Personal Food Policy – Food and Nutrition Services

F940 – Training Requirement – General – Training Requirements

F942 – Training Requirements – Resident's Rights Training

F947 – Training Requirements – Required In-Service Training for Nurse Aides

F948 – Required Training for Feeding Assistants – Training Requirements

F-tags for the Directors of Nursing

F725 – Sufficient Nursing Staff – Nursing Services

F726 – Competent Nursing Staff – Nursing Services

F727 – RN 8 Hrs./7 days/Wk., Full Time DON

F550 – Resident Rights/Exercise of Rights – Resident Rights

F561 – Self Determination – Resident Rights

F635 – Admissions Physician Orders for Immediate Care – Resident Assessments

F675 – Quality of Life – Quality of Life

F676 – Activities of Daily Living (ADLs)/Maintain Abilities – Quality of Life

F677 – ADL Care Provided for Dependent Residents – Quality of Life

F684 – Quality of Care – Quality of Care

F692 – Nutrition/Hydration Status Maintenance – Quality of Care

F810 – Assistive Devices – Eating Equipment/Utensils – Food and Nutrition Services

F811 – Feeding Asst.-Training/Supervision/Resident – Food and Nutrition Services

F813 – Personal Food Policy – Food and Nutrition Services

F947 – Required In-Service Training for Nurse Aides – Training Requirements

F948 – Training for Feeding Assistants – Training Requirements

F-tags for Dietitians

F800 – Provided Diet Meets Needs of Each Resident – Food and Nutrition Services

F801 – Qualified Dietary Staff – Food and Nutrition Services

F803 – Menus Meet Res Needs/Prep in Advance/Followed – Food and Nutrition Services

F805 – Food in Form to Meet Individual Needs (Food and Drink) – Food and Nutrition Service

F806 – Resident Allergies, Preferences and Substitutes – Food and Nutrition Services

F807 – Drinks Avail to Meet Needs/Preferences/Hydration – Food and Nutrition Services

F808 – Therapeutic Diet Prescribed by Physician – Food and Nutrition Services

F809 – Frequency of Meals/Snacks at Bedtime – Food and Nutrition Services

F813 – Personal Food Policy – Food and Nutrition Services

F675 – Quality of Life – Quality of Life

F684 – Quality of Care – Quality of Care

F692 – Nutrition/Hydration Status Maintenance – Quality of Care

F-tags for the Food Service Director/Manager

F800 – Provided Diet Meets Needs of Each Resident – Food and Nutrition Services

F801 – Qualified Dietary Staff – Food and Nutrition Services

F802 – Sufficient Dietary Support Personnel – Food and Nutrition Services

F803 –Menus Meet Res Needs/Prep in Advance/Followed – Food and Nutrition Services

F804 Nutritive Value/Appear, Palatable/Prefer Temp – Food and Nutrition Services

F805 – Food in Form to Meet Individual Needs – Food and Nutrition Services

F806 – Resident Allergies, Preferences and Substitutes – Food and Nutrition Services

F807 – Drinks Avail to Meet Needs/Preferences/Hydration – Food and Nutrition Services

F808 – Therapeutic Diet Prescribed by Physician – Food and Nutrition Services

F809 – Frequency of Meals/Snacks at Bedtime – Food and Nutrition Services

F810 – Assistive Devices–Eating Equipment/Utensils – Food and Nutrition Services

F812 – Food Procurement, Store/Prepare/Serve–Sanitary – Food and Nutrition Services

F813 – Personal Food Policy – Food and Nutrition Services

F814 – Dispose of Garbage & Refuse Properly – Food and Nutrition Services

F675 – Quality of Life – Quality of Life

F684 – Quality of Care – Quality of Care

F692 – Nutrition/Hydration Status Maintenance – Quality of Care

F-tags for Nurse Managers and Certified Nurse Aides or Certified Nursing Assistants thru the Director of Nursing

F550 – Resident Rights/Exercise of Rights – Resident Rights

F561 – Self Determination – Resident Rights

F584 – Safe/Clean/Comfortable/Homelike Environment – Resident Rights

F635 – Admission Physician Orders for Immediate Care – Resident Assessments

F636 – Comprehensive Assessments & Timing – Resident Assessment

F637 – Comprehensive Assessments & Timing – Resident Assessment

F641 – Accuracy of Assessments – Resident Assessments

F655 – Baseline Care Plan – Comprehensive Resident Centered Care Plans

F656 – Develop/Implement Comprehensive Care Plan – Comprehensive Resident Centered Care Plan

F657 – Care Plan Timing and Revision – Comprehensive Resident Centered Care Plans

F675 – Quality of Life – Quality of Life

F676 – Activities of Daily Living (ADLs)/Maintain Abilities – Quality of Life

F677 – ADL Care Provided for Dependent Residents – Quality of Life

F684 – Quality of Care – Quality of Care

F692 – Nutrition/Hydration Status Maintenance – Quality of Care

F693 – Tube Feeding Management/Restore Eating Skills – Quality of Care

F725 – Sufficient Nursing Staff – Nursing Services

F726 – Competent Nursing Staff – Nursing Services

F727 – RN 8 Hrs/7 days/Wk, Full Time DON – Nursing Services

F728 – Facility Hiring and Use of Nurse Aide – Nursing Services

F729 Nurse Aide Registry Verification, Retraining – Nursing Services

F807 – Drinks Avail to Meet Needs/Preferences/Hydration – Food and Nutrition Services

F808 – Therapeutic Diet Prescribed by Physician – Food and Nutrition Services

F809 – Frequency of Meals/Snacks at Bedtime – Food and Nutrition Services

F810 – Assistive Devices-Eating Equipment/Utensils – Food and Nutrition Services

F947 – Required In-Service Training for Nurse Aides – Training Requirements

F948 – Training of Feeding Assistants – Training Requirements

F949 – Behavioral health

F-tags for All Departments

F865 - Quality Assurance Performance Improvement (QAPI)

F867 – QAPI - Program feedback, data system, monitoring, systemic action

PART

3

Chapter 4

ADMINISTRATORS ROLE AND F-TAG FOCUS

Questions for Administrators

As the administrator you have the responsibility for the overall management of your SNF. It is the expectation that you are aware of what goes on in your facility. And how do you as the administrator accomplish this awesome task? Having broad knowledge of the regulations is important, determining and deciphering the important issues and matters that require your direct involvement is important, determining what needs to be delegated to your department directors is also important, and maintaining a culture of trust, respect, integrity and teamwork to name a few of the values, with department directors is also very essential.. You are the role model for your facility.

Here are self-assessment questions that I recommend you reflect on and answer as self-assessment. You can discuss and get feedback from colleagues if your so wish. There are seven (7) questions for self-assessment. You can use the blank spaces after each question for your objective evaluation and assessment of yourself as best as you can. Assess where you think you are and where you want you and your facility to be in order to meet your residents' needs as well as, your staffs' needs.

Questions for Administrators:

1. What culture and environment have you established for your facility, and what type of culture do you think your staff would say they are working in?

2. CMS has placed such a focus on staff competencies, and also on ensuring that facilities engage in consistent monitoring for quality, how will you grade your facility in meeting these expectations at your facility? (from 1 to 10, with 1 the lowest and 10 the highest)

3. One of the major challenges in the long term care industry is change; it is revision of regulations and new CMS Memoranda, requiring facilities update and revise standards or regulations. How do you and members of your team stay abreast of new memorandum issued by CMS to make sure that Quality of Care and Services are sustained and maintained?

4. Do you participate periodically or regularly in the "Environmental of Care Rounds" or in the monitoring of the "Resident Mealtime Experience"? And do also participate in daily rounds to the units?

5. How well do you know the regulations pertinent to Administrator's role and responsibilities for the efficient running of your facility and for the quality of resident care and services?

6. On a scale of 1 to 10, with 1 being the least prepared and 10 being the most prepared, how will you grade your facility's preparation for the upcoming Federal or State survey?

7. You are aware that when surveyors walk through your doors, they observe resident meal time on day one of the survey, are your Nurse Managers aware of this fact and how well do they participate in resident's mealtime monitoring?

F-tags Focus for Administrators

Below are F-tags that cover some of the areas of your responsibilities as administrators and leaders in your facilities. The overall management of the facility depends on you and your team. How well the staffs provide quality of care and services for residents, the quality of life that the residents need and deserves, the pleasant mealtime experience that contributes to the quality of life for the residents, resident safety, and also the healthy work environment you establish for your staffs, all lead to an effective and successful facility operation. CMS mandates that administrators must use the resources of the facility efficiently and effectively.

As stated, these F-Tags are from the current Centers for Medicare & Medicaid Services (CMS) State Operations Manual Appendix PP – Guidance to Surveyors for Long Term Care Facilities (Rev. 211; 02-03-23).

The F-tags, INTENT and DEFINITIONS, that I have listed in this workbook carry the regulatory language as stated in the State Operations Manual (SOM). For the **GUIDANCE** for most of the F-tags I included an abridged form of the regulatory language of the GUIDANCE. The guidance for some of the f-tags have detailed content, and I included that you need to refer to the State Operations Manual for the full content. Also for some of the F-tags you will see "**Remarks**" which I inserted, as needed for me to shed additional focus on certain points of the regulation and guidance to surveyors.

F-Tags:
F835
(Rev. 173, Issued: 11-22-17, Effective: 11-28-17, Implementation: 11-28-17)
§483.70 Administration.

A facility must be administered in a manner that enables it to use its resources effectively and efficiently to attain or maintain the highest practicable physical, mental, and psychosocial well-being of each resident.

GUIDANCE §483.70

Resources include but not limited to a facility's operating budget, staff, supplies, or other services necessary to provide for the needs of residents.

F836
(Rev. 173, Issued: 11-22-17, Effective: 11-28-17, Implementation: 11-28-17
§483.70(a) Licensure.
A facility must be licensed under applicable State and Local Laws.
§483.70(b) Compliance with Federal, State, and Local Laws and Professional Standards.
The facility must operate and provide services in compliance with all applicable Federal, State, and local laws, regulations, and codes, and with accepted professional standards and principles that apply to professionals providing services in such a facility.

§483.70(c) Relationship to Other HHS Regulations

In addition to compliance with the regulations set forth in this subpart, facilities are obliged to meet the applicable provisions of other HHS regulations., including but not limited to those pertaining to nondiscrimination of the basis of race, color, or national origin (45 CFR part 80); nondiscrimination on the basis of disability (45 CFR part 84); nondiscrimination of the basis of age (45 CFR part 91); nondiscrimination on the basis of race, color, national origin, sex, age, or disability (45 CFR part 92); protection of human subjects of research (45 CFR part 46); and fraud and abuse (42 CFR part 455) and protection of individually identifiable health information (45 CFR parts 160 and 164). Violations of such other provisions may result in finding of non-compliance with this paragraph.

DEFINITIONS §483.70(a)-(c)

"Accepted professional standards and principles" means Federal, State and local laws or professional licensure standards.

An **"authority having jurisdiction"** is the public agency, i.e. Federal, State or local, or official(s) having the authority to make a determination of noncompliance, and is responsible for providing and signing official correspondence notifying the facility or professional of their final adverse action.

F550
(Rev. 173, Issued: 11-22-17, Effective: 11-28-17, Implementation: 11-28-17)
§483.10(a) Resident Rights

The resident has the right to a dignified existence, self-determination, and communication with and access to persons and services inside and outside the facility, including those specified in this section.

§483.10(a)(1) A facility must treat each resident with respect and dignity and care for each resident in a manner and in an environment that promotes maintenance or enhancement of his or her quality of life, recognizing each resident's individuality. The facility must protect and promote the rights of the resident.

§483.10(a)(2) A facility must provide equal access to quality care regardless of diagnosis, severity of condition, or payment source. A facility must establish and maintain identical policies and practices regarding transfer, discharge, and the provision of services under the State plan for all residents regardless of payment source.

§483.10(b) Exercise of Rights

The resident has the right to exercise his or her rights as a resident of the facility and as a citizen or resident of the United States.

§483.10(b)(1) The facility must ensure that the resident can exercise his or her rights without interference, coercion, discrimination, or reprisal from the facility.

§483.10(b)(2) The resident has the right to be free of interference, coercion, discrimination, and reprisal from the facility in exercising his or her rights and to be supported by the facility in the exercise of his or her rights as required under this subpart.

INTENT §483.10(a)-(b)(1)&(2)

All residents have rights guaranteed to them under Federal and State laws and regulations. This regulation is intended to lay the foundation for the resident rights requirements in long-term care facilities. Each resident has the right to be treated with dignity and respect. All activities and interactions with residents by any staff, temporary agency staff or volunteers must focus on assisting the resident in maintaining and enhancing his or her self-esteem and self-worth and incorporating the resident's, goals, preferences, and choices. When providing care and services, staff must respect each resident's individuality, as well as honor and value their input.

GUIDANCE §483.10(a)-(b)(1)&(2) (This is an abridged form of the guidance; refer to the State Operations Manual Appendix PP for Guidance to Surveyors for Long Term Care Facilities, for the full content of the guidance.)

Examples of treating residents with dignity and respect include, but not limited to:

- Encouraging and assisting residents to dress in their own clothes, rather than hospital-type gowns, and appropriate footwear for the time of day and individual preferences;
- Placing labels on each resident's clothing in a way that is inconspicuous and respects his or her dignity (for example, placing labeling on the inside of shoes and clothing or using a color coding system)
- Promoting resident independence and dignity while dining, such as avoiding
  - Daily use of disposable cutlery and dishware;
  - Bibs or clothing protectors instead of napkins (except by resident choice);
  - Staff standing over residents while assisting them to eat;
  - Staff interacting/conversing only with each other rather than with residents while assisting with meals
- Protecting and valuing residents' private space (for example, knocking on doors and requesting permission before entering, closing doors as requested by the resident);

Remarks:

Remarks - I will recommend to Administrators, that you make "Resident Rights" frequent in-services in your facility for all staff. In addition to the regular staff competency sessions by Staff Development, you can include this topic in your General Staff Meetings and also have your Director of Nursing and Nurse Managers include this topic in their monthly staff meetings also. Disrespect and lack of sensitivity to resident rights leads facilities to receive visits from the Ombudsman and also to undergo "Complaint Surveys", as disrespect to residents must not be tolerated.

In the GUIDANCE section, recommendation is that staff must encourage residents to dress in their own clothes rather than in hospital gowns. As the focus is on quality and on resident mealtime experience, the goal for facility staffs must be to maintain a pleasant dining and mealtime experience for the residents, which has been stressed is part of quality of life. The staffs must treat the residents as individuals, in a person-centered manner recognizing their preferences and choices. While residents are eating in the dining room, staffs must also not be interacting talking loudly to each other while the residents are eating their meals.

F584
(Rev. 211; Issued: 02-03-23; Effective:10-21-22; Implementation: 10-24-22)
§483.10(i) Safe Environment

The resident has a right to a safe, clean, comfortable and homelike environment, including but not limited to receiving treatment and supports for daily living safely.

The facility must provide—

§483.10(i)(1) A safe, clean, comfortable, and homelike environment, allowing the resident to use his or her personal belongings to the extent possible.

   (i)   **This includes ensuring that the resident can receive care and services safely and That the physical layout of the facility maximizes resident independence and does not pose a safety risk.**

   (ii)   **The facility shall exercise reasonable care for the protection of the resident's property from loss or theft.**

§483.10(i)(2) Housekeeping and maintenance services necessary to maintain sanitary, orderly, and comfortable interior;

§483.10(i)(3) Clean bed and bath linens that are in good condition;

§483.10(i)(4) Private closet space in each resident room, as specified in §483.90(e)(2)(iv)

§483.10(5) Adequate and comfortable lighting levels in all areas;

§483.10(i)(6) Comfortable and safe temperature levels. Facilities initially certified after October 1, 1990 must maintain a temperature range 71 to 81 F

§483.10(i)(7) For the maintenance of comfortable sound levels.

DEFINITIONS §483.10(i)

"Adequate lighting" means levels of illumination suitable to tasks the resident chooses to perform or the facility staff must perform.

"Comfortable lighting" means lighting that minimizes glare and provide maximum resident control, where feasible, over the intensity, location, and direction of lighting to meet their needs or enhance independent functioning.

"Comfortable and safe temperature levels" means that the ambient temperature should be in a relatively narrow range that maintain residents' susceptibility to loss of body heat and risk of hypothermia, or hyperthermia, or and is comfortable for the residents.

"Comfortable sound levels" do not interfere with resident's hearing and enhance privacy when privacy is desired, and encouraged interaction when social participation is desired. Of particular concern to comfortable sound levels is the resident's control over unwanted noise.

"Environment" refers to any environment in the facility that is frequented by residents, including (but not limited to) the residents' rooms, bathrooms, hallways, dining areas, lobby, outdoor patios, therapy areas and activity areas.

A **"homelike environment"** is one that de-emphasizes the institutional character of the setting, to the extent possible, and allows the resident to use those personal belongings that support a homelike environment. A determination of "homelike" should include the resident's opinion of the living environment.

"Orderly" is defined as an uncluttered physical environment that is neat and well-kept.

"Sanitary" includes, but is not limited to, preventing the spread of disease-causing organisms by keeping resident care equipment clean and properly stored.. Resident care equipment includes, but is not limited to, equipment used in the completion of the activities of daily living.

GUIDANCE §483.10(i) (Below is an abridged form of the guidance; refer to the State Operations Manual Appendix PP for the full content of the guidance)

The concept of creating a home setting includes the elimination of institutional odors, and practices to the extent possible. Some practices that can be eliminated to decrease the institutional character of the environment include, but are not limited to, the following:

- Overhead paging (including frequent announcements) and piped-in music throughout the building.
- Meal service using trays (some residents may wish to eat certain meals on trays)
- Institutional signs labeling work rooms/closets in areas visible to residents and the public.
- The widespread and long-term use of audible chair and bed alarms, instead of their limited use for selected residents for diagnostic purposes or according to their care planned needs.
- Furniture that does not reflect a home-like environment or is uncomfortable; the absence of window treatments or drapes.

F675
(Rev. 211; Issued: 02-03-23; Effective: 10-21-22; Implementation: 10-24-22)
§483.24 Quality of Life

Quality of life is a fundamental principle that applies to all care and services provided to facility residents. Each resident must receive and the facility must provide the necessary care and services to attain or maintain the highest practicable physical, mental, and psychosocial well-being, consistent with the resident's comprehensive assessment and plan of care.

INTENT

The intent of this requirement is to specify the facility's responsibility to create and sustain an environment that humanizes and individualizes each resident's quality of life by:

- Ensuring all staff, across all shifts and departments, understand the principles of quality of life, and honor and support these principles for each resident; and
- Ensuring that the care and services provided are person-centered, and honor and support each resident's preferences, choices, values and beliefs.

DEFINITIONS §483.24

"Person Centered Care" – For the purposes of this subpart, person-centered care means to focus on the resident as the locus of control and support the resident in making their own choices and having control over their daily lives. (Definitions - §483.5)

"Pervasive" For the purposes of this guidance, pervasive means spread through or embedded within every part of something.

"Quality of Life" refers to an individual's "sense of well-being, level of satisfaction with life and feeling of self-worth and self-esteem. For nursing home residents, this includes a basic sense of satisfaction with oneself, the environment, the care received, the accomplishments of desired goals, and control over one's life." Adapted from the 1986 Institute of Medicine (IOM) published report "Improving the Quality of Care in Nursing Homes," located at: https://www.ncbi.nlm.nih.gov/books/NBK217548/#ddd00037"

GUIDANCE §483.24 (This is an abridge form of the guidance; refer to the State Operations Manual Appendix PP for the full content of the guidance)

Noncompliance at F675 identifies outcomes which rise to the level of immediate jeopardy and reflect an environment of pervasive disregard for the quality of life of the facility's residents. This can include the cumulative effect of noncompliance at other regulatory tags on one or more residents. To cite noncompliance at F675, the survey team must have evidence that outcomes at other regulatory tags demonstrate a pervasive disregard for the principles of quality of life.

Principles of Quality of Life (please note this is abridged. For complete version of this section, please refer to current State Operations Manual))

According to the 1986 Institute of Medicine (IOM) published report "Improving the Quality of Care in Nursing Homes," principles of Quality of Life included:

- A sense of well-being, satisfaction with life, and feeling of self-worth and self-esteem; and
- A sense of satisfaction with oneself, the environment, the care received the accomplishments of desired goals, and control over one's life.

F684
(Rev. 173, Issued: 11-22-17, Effective: 11-28-17, Implementation: 11-28-17)
§483.25 Quality of care

Quality of Care is fundamental principle that applies to all treatment and care provided to facility residents. Based on the comprehensive assessment of a resident, the facility must ensure that residents receive treatment and care in accordance with professional standards of practice, the comprehensive person-centered care plan, and the residents' choices, including but not limited to the following:

INTENT

To ensure facilities identify and provide needed care and services that are resident centered, in accordance with the resident's preferences, goals for care and professional standards of practice that will meet each resident's physical, mental, and psychosocial needs.

DEFINITIONS

"Highest practicable physical, mental, and psychosocial well-being" is defined as the highest possible level of functioning and well-being, limited by the individual's recognized pathology and normal aging process. Highest practicable is determined through the comprehensive resident assessment and by recognizing and completely and thoroughly addressing the physical, mental, and psychosocial needs of the individual.

"Hospice Care" means a comprehensive set of services described in Section 1861(dd)(1) of the Act, identified and coordinated by an interdisciplinary group (IDG) to provide for the physical, psychosocial, spiritual, and emotional needs of a terminally ill patient and/or family members, as delineated in a specific patient plan of care. (42 CFR §418.3)

"Palliative care" means patient and family-centered care that optimizes quality of life by anticipating, preventing, and treating suffering. Palliative care throughout the continuum of illness involves addressing physical, intellectual, emotional, social, and spiritual needs and to facilitate patient autonomy, access to information, and choice. (§418.3)

"Terminally ill" means that the individual has a medical prognosis that his or her life expectancy is 6 months or less if the illness runs its normal course. (§418.3)

GUIDANCE (This is an abridged form of the guidance ; refer to the State Operations Manual Appendix PP for the full content of the guidance)

Nursing homes must place priority on identifying what each resident's highest practicable well-being is in each of the areas of physical, mental and psychosocial health. Each resident's care plan must reflect person-centered care, and include resident choices, preferences, goals concerns/needs, and describe the services and care that is to be furnished to attain or maintain, or improve the resident's highest practicable physical, mental and psychosocial well-being. For concerns related to the resident's comprehensive care plan, see F656, §483.21(b) Comprehensive Care Plans.

F920
(Rev. 173, Issued: 11-22-17, Effective: 11-28-17, Implementation: 11-28-17)
§483.90(h) Dining and Resident Activities

The facility must provide one or more rooms designated for resident dining and activities.

These rooms must—

§483.90(h)(1) Be well lighted;
§483.90(h)(2) Be well ventilated;
§483.90(h)(3) Be adequately furnished; and
§483.90(h)(4) Have sufficient space to accommodate all activities.

GUIDANCE: §483.90(h)(1), (h)(2), (h)(3) and (h)(4)

"**Well lighted**" is defined as levels of illumination that are suitable to tasks performed by a resident.

"**Well ventilated**" is defined as good air circulation, avoidance of drafts at floor level, and adequate smoke and odor exhaust removal.

Reference ASHRAE Standard 179 for ventilation requirements in nursing homes activity and dining areas.

An "**adequately furnished**" dining area accommodates different residents' physical and social needs. An adequately furnished organized activities area accommodates the needs, interests and preferences of its residents.

"**Sufficient space to accommodate all activities**" means that there is enough space available and it is adaptable to a variety of uses and residents' needs.

F813
(Rev. 173, Issued: 11-22-17, Effective: 11-28-17, Implementation: 11-28-17)
§483.60(i) Food Safe Requirements

The facility must –

§483.60(i)(3) Have a policy regarding use and storage of foods brought to residents by family and other visitors to ensure safe and sanitary storage, handling, and consumption.

GUIDANCE §483.60(i)(3) (This is an abridged form of the guidance; refer to the State Operations Manual Appendix PP for the full content of the guidance)

The facility must have a policy regarding food brought to residents by family and other visitors. The policy must also include ensuring facility staff assists the resident in accessing and consuming the food, if the resident is not able to do so on his or her won. The facility also is responsible for storing food brought in by family or visitors in a way that is either separate or easily distinguishable from facility food.

The facility has responsibility to help family and visitors understand safe food handling practices (such as safe cooling/reheating processes, hot/cold holding temperatures, preventing cross contamination, hand hygiene, etc.) If the facility is assisting family or visitors with reheating or other preparation activities, facility staff must use safe food handling practices.

F940
(Rev. 211; Issued: 02-03-23; Effective: 10-21-22; Implementation: 10-24-22)
§483.95 Training Requirements

A facility must develop, implement, and maintain an effective training program for all new and existing staff; individuals providing services under a contractual arrangement; and volunteers, consistent with their expected roles. A facility must determine the amount and types of training necessary based on a facility assessment as specified at §483.70(e). Training topics must include but not limited to –

INTENT – (This is an abridged form of the intent; refer to the State Operations Manual- for full content of the intent)

Facilities are required to develop, implement, and maintain an effective training program for all staff. Appropriately trained staff can improve resident safety, create a more person-centered environment, and reduce the number of adverse events or other resident complications.

CMS recognizes that training needs are likely to change over time. Therefore, it is necessary for facilities to have the flexibility to determine training needs based on its facility assessment. Competencies and skill sets for all new and existing staff, individuals providing services under a contractual arrangement, and volunteers must be consistent with their expected roles. All facility staff needs to be trained to be able to interact in a manner that enhances the resident's quality of life and quality of care and that they can demonstrate competency in the topic areas of the training program. ......

F942
(Rev. 211: Issued 02-03-23; Effective: 10-21-22; Implementation: 10-24-22)
§483.95 Training Requirements

Training topics must include but not limited to

§483.95(b) Resident's rights and facility responsibilities.

A facility must ensure that staff members are educated on the rights of the resident and the responsibilities of a facility to properly care for its residents as set forth at §483.10, respectively.

INTENT

To ensure all facility staff understand and foster the rights of every nursing home resident. For the purpose of this training requirement, staff includes all facility staff, (direct and indirect care functions), contracted staff, and volunteers (training topics as appropriate to role.)

GUIDANCE §483.95(b) (This is an abridged form of the guidance refer to the State Operations Manual for the full content)

Facilities must develop and implement an ongoing education program on all resident rights and facility responsibilities for caring of residents as outlined in §483.10

The education program should support current scope and standards of practice through curricula which incorporate learning objectives, performance standards, and evaluation criteria. Staff performance assessments should evaluate the ability to integrate knowledge and skills specific to the requirements at §483.10

There should be a process in place to validate that training was completed, whether in a group setting or on an individual basis.

F947
"(Rev. 211; Issued: 02-03-23; Effective: 10-21-22; Implementation: 10-24-22)
§483.95 Training Requirements.

Training topics must include but not limited to—-

§483.95(g) Required in-service training for nurse aides.

In-service training must-----

§483.95(g)(1) Be sufficient to ensure the continuing competencies of nurse aides, but must be no less than 12 hours per year.

§483.95(g)(2) Include dementia management training and resident abuse prevention training.

§483.95(g)(3) Address areas of weakness as determined in nurse aides' performance reviews and facility assessment at §483.70(e) and may address the special needs of residents as determined by the facility staff.

§483.95(g)(4) For nurse aides providing services to individuals with cognitive impairments, also address the care of the cognitively impaired.

DEFINITIONS

A "**nurse aide**" is defined in §483.5 as any individual providing nursing or nursing-related services to residents in a facility. This term may also include an individual who provides these services through an agency or under a contract with the facility, but is not a licensed health professional, a registered dietitian, or someone who volunteers to provide such services without pay. Nurse aides do not include those individuals who furnish services to residents only as paid feeding assistants as defined in §488.301.

Private duty nurse aides who are not employed or utilized by the facility on a contract, per diem, leased, or other basis, do not come under the nurse aide training provision and therefore are not required to take the training.

Performance Reviews: The process used to evaluate the performance of staff on a periodic basis, which may be annually.

NOTE: See Tag F730-§483.35(d)(7) related to the conduct of performance reviews for every nurse aide at least once every 12 months.

For **GUIDANCE** – (refer to the State Operations Manual for the content)

F948
(Rev. 173, Issued: 11-22-17, Effective: 11-28-17, Implementation: 11-28-17)
§483.95(h) Required training of feeding assistants.

A facility must not use any individual working in the facility as paid feeding assistant unless that individual has successfully completed a State-approved training program for feeding assistants, as specified in §483.160.

DEFINITION §483.95(h)

Paid feeding assistant is defined in the regulation at 42 CFR 488.301 as "an individual who meets the requirements specified in §483.60(h)(1) of this chapter and who is paid to feed residents by a facility, or who is used under an arrangement with another agency or organization.

F949
(Rev. 211: Issued: 02-03-23; Effective: 10-21-22; Implementation: 10-24-22)
§483.95 Training Requirements

Training topics must include but not limited to--

§483.95(i) Behavioral health.

A facility must provide behavioral health training consistent with the requirements at §483.40 and as determined by the facility assessment at §483.70(e)

GUIDANCE §483.95(i) (This is abridged form of the guidance; refer to the State Operations Manual for the full content)

All facilities must develop, implement, and maintain an effective training program for all staff, which includes, at a minimum, training on behavioral health care and services (consistent with §483.40) that is appropriate and effective, as determined by staff need and the facility assessment (as specified at §483.70(e). For the purposes of this training requirement, staff includes all facility staff, (direct and indirect care functions), contracted staff, and volunteers (training topics as appropriate to role).

Changes to the facility's resident population, staff turnover, the facility's physical environment, and modifications to the facility assessment may require ongoing revisions to the facility's training program.

Chapter 5

PRACTICAL TIPS FOR ADMINISTRATORS AND CASE STUDY

Practical Tips

As much as long term care is a rewarding profession because you have the opportunity to impact lives in a positive way; there are challenges that come with the job and with the industry. Administrators, you have the ultimate responsibility to ensure that staffs provide quality of care, quality of life and safe environment for the residents, and the goal of meeting regulatory compliance. Concerning resident dining and mealtime experience, it has been established that mealtime contributes to the residents quality of life; inevitably you want make certain that the residents routinely have a pleasant mealtime experience while meeting their nutritional needs.

The environment in your facility should be one that enables your staffs at all level to demonstrate great customer service, quality of patient-care and service, an understanding of the concept of inter-relatedness of all departments and disciplines within the facility. With that understanding the concept of teamwork will flow together for a smooth running of the facility. Continuous quality and performance improvement is a must and you and your QAPI Director/Coordinator must work towards a robust and effective QAPI Program.

Below are tips to help you with the operation of your facility and may reduce some of the daily stress that comes with the job. The operations in all facilities may be different, so you utilize these tips based on your facility environment and your choice.

Tips for Administrators:

- The culture within the facility - As the administrator you are the leader and you want to develop an environment that is pleasant and positive, that is inviting as a good place for staff to work in. Of course you cannot do this alone by yourself, but as the leader you set the character and culture of what you want the facility to project. Review your organization's value statement to see if your facility is living up to the value statement. If not work with Human Resource Director and other department heads to plan strategic sessions to take corrective action for improvement of the facility's environment to match your organization's values.

- Teamwork – You cannot accomplish much without great teamwork; and teamwork starts with you. Your F-tag regulation requires you to manage and run the facility so your residents attain or maintain the highest practicable physical, mental, and psychosocial well-being. In order to accomplish this you must work well with your director of nursing, and both you and the director of nursing have to exhibit to the rest of the staff what teamwork looks like. Regularly scheduled department head meetings are a great contribution to teamwork within the facility.

- Mentoring - Mentor and help develop your department directors/department heads as best as you possibly can in areas and skills that they may be a little lacking. Management and supervisory skills are areas that they may need help.

- Communication – Communication is one of the keys to effective leadership and cohesive facility infrastructure and lack of communication leads to dysfunction. Everyone knows communication is very important and as the leader you need help make effective communication happen, in your facility. Listening is an important part of communication.

- Working Relationship with the Director of Nursing - Make your Director of Nursing your "right-hand woman or man". Let her, let him know how important they are, and that you appreciate the work they do. Work closely with your Director of Nursing (DON) to ensure that you are kept abreast of care issues that you need to know about.

- Resident Meal Time and Dining Experience - work closely with the DON and the Director of Food Service to ensure the residents receive the desired Quality of Life in this area, meeting their nutritional needs. Be intentional and ask questions. Increase your awareness of the roles and responsibilities of the Dietitian through the Food Service Director/Manager to ensure the residents' nutritional needs are routinely met, and that they have pleasant mealtime and dining experience.

- Clinical Meetings - It is important to make time to attend clinical meetings – you can determine how often you want to attend, but be present in some of the clinical meetings.. This gives you first-hand knowledge on some of the patient care issues, and quality issues.

- Homelike ambience and safety of residents - Make sure your dining rooms are equipped with homelike type dining furniture, and that Life Safety and environment of care standards are maintained.

- Daily Rounds – participate in rounds on the units; talk to staff and talk to residents. Determine how often you want to do rounds on the unit and how much time you want to allocate on daily rounds., I recommend daily if possible (five days a week). Making rounds on the unit for about an hour to an hour and a half daily helps your visibility in the facility and helps the residents, the families and the staffs know that you care about them, and this goes a long way towards the staff-administrator relationship and resident-administrator relationship.

- Be a problem solver – when problems are brought to your attention by your department heads, seek input from them and then help them solve the problems.

- Department Head Meetings - Establish weekly or bi-weekly Department Head meetings, where you and the team share updates of what is going on in their departments, and share and discuss ideas. Also set up monthly general staff meetings for all staffs.

- QAPI - Ensure your facility has an effective Quality Assurance Performance Improvement (QAPI) program. Have the monitoring for Resident Meal Time be part of the QAPI reporting schedule; and work closely with the DON, with QAPI to have regular monitoring of resident meal time experience. Your Infection Preventionist should be important member of the committee. This also helps make your facility survey ready.

- Environment of Care Rounds - Ensure your facility develops weekly "Environment of Care" Rounds, and you can participate with the team monthly. This helps your facility's survey readiness. Infection Preventionist should also be part of this team.

- Ensure your facility has an effective Staff Development Program for timely and required competencies for the staff. Make sure that required competencies for nursing department and food service staff are done regularly.

- Needed Resources - Make sure your facility has the available resources to manage the facility efficiently and effectively, and do not be hesitant to let your CEO or the District Director, or the Owner know what resources you need.

- Know your regulations as best as possible, not to memorize them but know when you need to refer to them for clarification, and be aware of what some of the "Best Practices" for long term care are and incorporate them within your facility's operations.

- Financial Viability of your Facility – of course you need to pay close attention to your monthly financial statements to review your profit and loss statements.. Have a system to monitor Admissions, Daily Census, Occupancy Rate, Case Mix, expenses, and financial statements and set up monthly meetings for financial reporting.

The case study below is for you to review and come up with the best solutions to resolve the issues. You can discuss with members of your team and brainstorm solutions. There are questions at the end of the case study and you can do the exercise alone or work together with your colleagues or the relevant department heads.

CASE STUDY:

As Administrators you have different situations and challenges that have happened at your facilities and I know that as often as you solve problems new problems arise.. Problem solving is a big part of your job, whether they are problems dealing with resident care, family dissatisfaction, or staff situations. This is part of the daily life of the administrator.

This case study does not reflect any specific situation(s) in any specific SNF or Nursing Home. Review the case study, and answer the questions that follow. Names used here for this case study are also fictitious names.

DISCLAIMER: The workbook case studies are fictional – fictional names of skilled nursing facilities and/or nursing homes, fictional situations and fictional stories. The names, characters and incidents portrayed in the case studies are fictional, and no identification with persons (living or dead) and with places or with products should be assumed or inferred.

CASE STUDY

On a beautiful Monday morning, the Administrator walked into his office prepared and ready to tackle his "To Do List". He told his Administrative Assistant, "Do you know, I have my To-Do list here and I received a call from one resident yesterday and I promised to see her first thing this morning. After my visit with Mrs. Reynolds, I will head over to my Department Head meeting, and after that, I will tackle the things on my to-do list. I hope nothing else happens, to take me away from plans for today. So if you can do me a favor, just take messages for me until I get back down to my office, so I can get these things done that I have on my list for today,"

As soon as the administrator was about ready to leave his office to go meet with the resident, the Admin. Assistant came in and told the administrator "Guess what, the resident's daughter is on the phone for you". The administrator obviously had to take that call. The Admin Assistant called the Nurse Manager on the unit asked her to let Resident know that the administrator will meet with her soon, that he had not forgotten the meeting that he had promised. The administrator took the call, and the daughter had a complaint about everything that transpired on Sunday concerning the dinner meal, as the resident had called her daughter about her meal time experience the previous day. Fortunately for the administrator, the nursing supervisor had also called him on Sunday and informed him of the situation about the resident's dinner meal experience, when the situation was happening..

After talking to the daughter, the administrator then went up to the unit to meet with the Resident, who also relayed the happenings of Sunday, and all the things that did not go well with her dinner meal.

The complaint centered this situation, when the resident who had been at ABC SNF for many months, when she became quite ill and her attending physician made a decision to send her to the hospital. She was transferred to the hospital based on doctor's orders and admitted at the hospital for four (4) days. The resident progressed, got better and was discharged back to the SNF. Prior to discharge, the discharge planner at the hospital called the SNF to let them know that the hospital team thinks the patient was ready to be discharged back to the SNF. Arrangements were made and the paperwork completed for the discharge. The patient went back to the SNF Sunday afternoon. Resident Mrs. Reynolds was well received by the SNF and made comfortable.

The problem arose when the resident was presented with a regular diet for dinner. The resident told the certified nurse aide, "Do you know that my diet was changed to mechanical soft diet, why do I have regular diet on my plate?'. The nurse aide informed the resident, "this is the diet that the kitchen sent up for you". The resident insisted that what she had on her plate was not her current diet. The nurse aide then summoned the nursing supervisor for resolution of the problem. The nursing supervisor who was in her office at that time, came to the dining room where the resident was with the wrong tray.. The supervisor and the nurse aide apologized to the resident and removed the dinner tray from the table, and told the resident that they would get her the correct diet, again apologizing to the resident. This became an unpleasant situation for the resident, as everyone in the dinning within earshot had the conversation going on, and the resident did not have her meal at the time everyone else were eating their meal. This was a very unpleasant experience for the resident. She called her daughter to inform her of this meal time experience.

What are the service recovery steps the facility needs to take or should have taken, and moving forward what system will the administrator and his team put in place to make sure that situation or any similar situation does not happen again? See questions below on "Exercises to Do" for service recovery. You can add to the questions as you see fit.

Exercises to Do

As the Administrator, how will you handle the Service Recovery here?

The most important hint is "Do not blame the people (staffs), look at your system.

A. What is the first step that the administrator should take?

B. Which Team Members need to review the current system? Note: You cannot fix the problem until you review your current system.

C. List potential solutions to address and fix the system

D. What monitoring will you put in place for new admissions and re-admissions coming to your facility so the required disciplines and staffs are aware of any diet changes?

E. What is the Quality Assurance and Performance Improvement (QAPI)'s role and responsibility in this situation? Moving forward - What do you expect from the QAPI Director/Manager/Coordinator and other members of the team?

F. When you report back to the resident and to her daughter, what do you think you will say and how do you feel your response will be received?

PART
4

Chapter 6

DIRECTORS OF NURSING ROLE AND F-TAG FOCUS

Questions for Directors of Nursing and F-Tags Focus

As Directors of Nursing you have overall responsibility for the Nursing Department and clinical nursing care for the residents. You are the direct supervisors for the Nurse Managers, Charge Nurses, Direct Care licensed nurses, who are supervisors for certified Nurse Aides or Certified Nursing Assistants, and other nursing related staff.. You must work collaboratively with other Department Directors and Department Heads, including the Administrator and the Medical Director. The Nursing discipline and other disciplines such as Rehabilitative Services, Social Work Services, Dietitian, Therapeutic Recreation Services, Minimum Data Set (MDS). You have a key role to play working with the licensed nurses and the Interdisciplinary Team to ensure residents are assessed upon admission, that 48-Hour care plan and future care plans are developed and implemented throughout the residents' stay in the facility.

As stated above, in addition to working closely with the medical director, your role and responsibility also demands that you work collaboratively with attending physicians and physician extenders to ensure residents Quality of Care and Services, Quality of Life and resident safety are maintained. It is essential that the Administrator and the Director of Nursing have a very good working relationship for smooth running of the facility.

These questions for Directors of Nursing will give you an opportunity to review and assess how well you are doing in these areas. I am leaving blank spaces between questions for you to pen down your answers.

Questions for Director of Nursing

1. How well do you work with the administrator and the medical director to ensure that the residents receive Quality of Care and Services, Quality of Life and Safety in your facility?

2. How well do you work with the dietitian and food service director/manager to ensure that the residents nutritional needs are met, and that the residents have pleasant mealtime experience?

3. How do you ensure that the licensed nurses, nurse aides and other related nursing staff maintain their required competencies to enhance their clinical skill sets?

4. Do you conduct daily (Monday thru Friday) clinical meetings with your nurse managers and members of the other disciplines to discuss residents' clinical conditions, including the newly admitted residents; and data that need to be reviewed?

5. Residents change in condition and residents readmissions to the hospital – what systems do you have in place to monitor for potential to address these clinical issues as necessary?

6. How well do you know the regulations for nursing and other regulations that impact nursing and patient/resident care, to ensure that the residents live up to their highest practicable physical, mental, and psychosocial well-being?

7. Will your residents say they are receiving the quality of care and Services, and quality of life?

8. How often and how well do you mentor your nurse managers, your nursing supervisors, and charge nurses to help them improve their supervisory skills and problem solving skills sets?

Below are the specific F-Tags for the Director of Nursing and Nursing Department. Just to remind you that these F-tags are also from the current State Operations Manual Appendix PP, with Revision date of 02-03-23.

F-Tags for Directors of Nursing

I have listed the F-Tags in order of priority not necessarily in numerical order or sequence. The **F-tags, the INTENT and DEFINITIONS** carry the language of the regulations. The guidance mostly are in abridged form. And I recommend that you refer to the State Operations Manual for the full content of the guidance. You will notice "**remarks**" which highlight certain areas I believe you also need to pay close attention to.

F-Tags
F725 -
(Rev. 211; Issued: 02-03-23; Effective:10-21-22; Implementation:10-24-22)
§483.35 Nursing Services

The facility must have sufficient nursing staff with the appropriate competencies and skills sets to provide nursing and related services to assure resident safety and attain or maintain the highest practicable physical, mental, and psychosocial well-being of each resident, as determined by resident assessments and individual plans of care and considering the number, acuity and diagnoses of the facility's resident population in accordance with the facility assessment required at §483.70(e).

§483.35(a) Sufficient Staff.

§483.35(a)(1)The facility must provide services by sufficient numbers of each of the following types of personnel on a 24-hour basis to provide nursing care to all residents in accordance with resident care plans:

(i)	**Except when waived under paragraph (e) of this section, licensed nurses; and**
(ii)	**Other nursing personnel, including but not limited to nurse aides.**

§483.35(a)(2) Except when waived under paragraph [(e)] of this section, the facility must designate a licensed nurse to serve as a charge nurse on each tour of duty.

INTENT §483.35(a)(1)-(2)

To assure that there is sufficient qualified nursing staff available at all times to provide nursing and related services to meet the residents' needs safely and in a manner that promotes each resident's rights, physical, mental and psychosocial well-being.

DEFINITIONS §§483.35(a)(1)-(2)

"**Nurse Aide**" as defined in §483.5, is any individual providing nursing or nursing-related services to residents in a facility. This term may also include an individual who provides these services through an agency or under a contract with the facility, but is not a licensed health professional, a registered dietitian, or someone who volunteers to provide such services without pay. Nurse aides do not include those individuals who furnish services to residents only as paid feeding assistants as defined in §488.301.

GUIDANCE §483.35(a)(1)-(2) (This is an abridged form of the guidance; refer to the State Operations Manual Appendix PP for Guidance to Surveyors for Long Term Care Facilities, for the full content of the guidance)

Many factors must be considered when determining whether or not a facility has sufficient staff to care for residents' needs, as identified through the facility assessment, resident assessments, and as described in their plan of care. A staffing deficiency under this requirement may or may not be directly related to an adverse outcome to a resident's care or services. It may also include the potential for physical or psychosocial harm.

As required under Administration at F838, §483.70(e) an assessment of the resident population is the foundation of the facility assessment and determination of the level of sufficient staff needed. It must include an evaluation of diseases, conditions, physical or cognitive limitations of the resident population's, acuity (the level of severity of residents' illnesses, physical, mental and cognitive limitations and conditions) and any other pertinent information about the resident population should drive staffing decisions and inform the facility about what skills and competencies staff must possess in order to deliver the necessary care required by the residents being served.

Remarks

Remarks - : CMS has added new information about facilities responsibilities to submit information on the facilities staffing. The additional information stresses the fact that facilities meeting their State minimum staffing requirement standard may not necessarily meet the Federal standards for staffing. As of this writing, it is required that facilities must provide licensed nursing staff 24 hours a day 7 days a week. CMS also is recommending to surveyors to probe and interview directors of nursing, administrators, and staff particularly if there are negative outcomes at the facility. Negative outcomes such as frequent falls, weight loss, dehydration, pressure ulcers could be an indication of not enough staff. There is a list of probing questions for surveyors to utilize when they interview facility staff. Please refer to the current State Operations Manual for more detailed information.

F726
(Rev. 173, Issued: 11-22-17, Effective: 11-28-17, Implementation: 11-28-17)
§483.35 Nursing Services

The facility must have sufficient nursing staff with the appropriate competencies and skills sets to provide nursing and related services to assure resident safety and attain or maintain the highest practicable physical, mental, and psychosocial well-being of each resident, as determined by resident assessments and individual plans

of care and considering the number, acuity and diagnoses of the facility's resident population in accordance with the facility assessment required at §483.70(e).

§483.35(a)(3) "The facility must ensure that licensed nurses have the specific competencies and skill sets necessary to care for residents' needs, as identified through resident assessments, and described in the plan of care.

§483.35(a)(4) Providing care includes but is not limited to assessing, evaluating, planning and implementing resident care plans and responding to resident's needs.

§483.35(c) Proficiency of nurse aides.

The facility must ensure that nurse aides are able to demonstrate competency in skills and techniques necessary to care for residents' needs, as identified through resident assessments, and described in the plan of care.

INTENT §483.35(a)(3)-(4),(c)

To assure that all nursing staff possess the competencies and skill sets necessary to provide nursing and related services to meet the residents' needs safely and in a manner that promotes each resident's rights, physical, mental and psychosocial well-being.

DEFINITIONS

"Competency" is a measurable pattern of knowledge, skills, abilities, behaviors, and other characteristics that an individual needs to perform work roles or occupational functions successfully.

F727
(Rev. 211: Issued: 02-03-23; Effective: 10-21-22; Implementation: 10-24-22)
§483.35(b) Registered nurse

§483.35(b)(1) Except when waived under paragraph (e) or (f) of this section, the facility must use the services of a registered nurse for at least 8 consecutive hours a day, 7 days a week.

§483.35(b)(2) Except when waived under paragraph (e) or (f) of this section, the facility must designate a registered nurse to serve as the director of nursing on a full time basis.

§483.35(b)(3) The director of nursing may serve as a charge nurse only when the facility has an average daily occupancy of 60 or fewer residents.

DEFINITIONS §483.35(b)

"Full time" is defined as working 40 or more hours a week.

"Charge Nurse" is a licensed nurse with specific responsibilities designated by the facility that may include staff supervision, emergency coordinator, physician liaison, as well as direct resident care.

PROCEDURES AND GUIDANCE §483.35(b) (This is an Abridged version of the GUIDANCE. CMS has added detailed new information on this GUIDANCE so I recommend you refer to the State Operations Manual Appendix PP for full content of the guidance)

PROCEDURES AND GUIDANCE §483.35(b)

Nurse staffing in nursing homes has a substantial impact on the quality of care and outcomes that residents experience. A registered nurse (RN) is typically responsible for overseeing the care provided to nursing home residents by other staff such as Licensed Practical Nurses (LPN) or Certified Nurse Aides (CNA). The RN is generally responsible for more advanced care activities such as resident assessments, consulting with physicians, and administering intravenous fluids or medications.

Facilities are responsible for ensuring they have an RN providing services at least 8 consecutive hours a day, 7 days a week. However, per Facility Assessment requirements at F838, §483.70(e), facilities are expected to identify when they may require the services of an RN for more than 8 hours a day based on the acuity level of the resident population. If it is determined the services of an RN are required for more than 8 hours a day, refer to the guidance at F725 related to sufficient nurse staffing for further investigation.

F550
(Rev. 173, Issued: 11-22-17, Effective: 11-28-17, Implementation: 11-28-17)
§483.10(a) Resident Rights.

The resident has a right to a dignified existence, self-determination, and communication with and access to persons and services inside and outside the facility, including those specified in this section.

§483.10(a)(1) A facility must treat each resident with respect and dignity and care for each resident in a manner and in an environment that promotes maintenance or enhancement of his or her quality of life, recognizing each resident's individuality. The facility must protect and promote the rights of the resident.

§483.10(a)(2) The facility must provide equal access to quality care regardless of diagnosis, severity of condition, or payment source. A facility must establish and maintain identical policies and practices regarding transfer, discharge, and the provision of services under the State plan for all residents regardless of payment source.

§483.10(b) Exercise of Rights.

The resident has the right to exercise his or her rights as a resident of the facility and as a citizen or resident of the United States.

§483.10(b)(1) The facility must ensure that the resident can exercise his or her rights without interference, coercion, discrimination, or reprisal from the facility.

§483.10(b)(2) The resident has the right to be free of interference, coercion, discrimination, and reprisal from the facility in exercising his or her rights and to be supported by the facility in the exercise of his or her rights as required under this subpart.

INTENT §483.10(a)-(b)(1)&(2)

All residents have rights guaranteed to them under Federal and State laws and regulations. This regulation is intended to lay the foundation for the resident rights requirements in long-term care facilities. Each resident has the right to be treated with dignity and respect. All activities and interactions with residents by any staff, temporary agency staff or volunteers must focus on assisting the resident in maintaining and enhancing his or her self-esteem and self-worth and incorporating the resident's, goals, preferences, and choices. When providing care and services, staff must respect each resident's individuality, as well as honor and value their input.

GUIDANCE §483.10(a)-(b)(1)&(2) This is an abridged form of the guidance.; refer to the State Operations Manual Appendix PP for the full content of the guidance)

Examples of treating residents with dignity and respect include, but are not limited to:

- Encouraging and assisting residents to dress in their own clothes, rather than hospital-type gowns, and appropriate footwear for the time of day and individual preferences;
- Placing labels on each resident's clothing in a way that is inconspicuous and respects his or her dignity (for example, placing labeling on the inside of shoes and clothing or using a color coding system);
- Promoting resident independence and dignity while dining, such as avoiding:
  - o Daily use of disposable cutlery and dishware;
  - o Bibs or clothing protectors instead of napkins (except by resident choice);
  - o Staff standing over residents while assisting them to eat;
  - o Staff interacting/conversing only with each other rather than with residents while assisting with meals.
- Protecting and valuing residents' private space (for example, knocking on doors and requesting permission before entering, closing doors as requested by the resident);

F561
(Rev. 211; Issued: 02-03-23; Effective: 10-21-22; Implementation: 10-24-22)
§483.10(f) Self-determination.

The resident has the right to and the facility must promote and facilitate resident self-determination through support of resident choice, including but not limited to the rights specified in paragraphs (f)(1) through (11) of this section.

§483.10(f)(1) The resident has a right to choose activities, schedules (including sleeping and waking times), health care and providers of health care services consistent with his or her interests, assessments, and plan of care and other applicable provisions of this part.

§483.10(f)(2) The resident has a right to make choices about aspects of his or her life in the facility that are significant to the resident.

§483.10(f)(3) The resident has a right to interact with members of the community and participate in community activities both inside and outside the facility.

§483.10(f)(8) The resident has a right to participate in other activities, including social, religious, and community activities that do not interfere with the rights of other residents in the facility.

INTENT §483.10(f)(1)-(3) and (8)

The intent of this requirement is to ensure that each resident has the opportunity to exercise his or her autonomy regarding those things that are important in his or her life. This includes the residents' interests and preferences.

GUIDANCE §483.10(f)(1)-)(3), (8) (This is an abridged form of the guidance, refer to the State Operations Manual Appendix PP for the full content of the guidance)

Residents have the right to choose their schedules, consistent with their interests, assessments, and care plans. This includes, but not limited to, choices about the schedules that are important to the resident, such as waking, eating, bathing, and going to bed at night. Choices about schedules and ensuring that residents are able to get enough sleep is an important contributor to overall health and well-being.

F635
(Rev. 173, Issued: 11-22-17, Effective: 11-28-17, Implementation: 11-28-17)
§483.20(a) Admissions orders

At the time each resident is admitted, the facility must have physician orders for the resident's immediate care.

INTENT §483.20(a)

To ensure each resident receives necessary care and services upon admission.

GUIDANCE §483.20(a)

"Physician orders for immediate care" are those written and/or verbal orders facility staff need to provide essential care to the resident, consistent with the resident's mental and physical status upon admission to the facility. These orders should, at a minimum, include dietary, medications (if necessary) and routine care to maintain or improve the resident's functional abilities until staff can conduct a comprehensive assessment and develop an interdisciplinary care plan.

F675
(Rev. 211, Issued: 02-03-23; Effective: 10-21-22; Implementation: 10-24-22)
§483.24 Quality of life

Quality of life is a fundamental principle that applies to all care and services provided to facility residents. Each resident must receive and the facility must provide the necessary care and services to attain or maintain the highest practicable physical, mental, and psychosocial well-being, consistent with the resident's comprehensive assessment and plan of care.

INTENT

The intent of this requirement is to specify the facility's responsibility to create and sustain an environment that humanizes and individualizes each resident's quality of life by:

- Ensuring all staff, across all shifts and departments, understand the principles of quality of life, and honor and support these principles for each resident; and
- Ensuring that the care and services provided are person-centered, and honor and support each resident's preferences, choices, values and beliefs.

DEFINITIONS §483.24"Person Centered Care" – For the purposes of this subpart, person-centered means to focus on the resident as the locus of control and support the resident in making their own choices and having control over their daily lives. (Definitions - §483.5)

"Pervasive" For the purposes of this guidance, pervasive means spread through or embedded within every part of something.

"Quality of Life" refers to an individual's "sense of well-being, level of satisfaction with life and feeling of self-worth and self-esteem. For nursing home residents, this includes a basic sense of satisfaction with oneself, the environment, the care received, the accomplishments of desired goals, and control over one's life." Adapted from the 1986 Institute of Medicine (IOM) published report "Improving the Quality of Care in Nursing Homes," located at: https://www.nchi.nlm.nih.gov/books/NBK217548/#ddd00037

(For **GUIDANCE** refer to the State operations Manual Appendix PP for full content of the guidance)

F676
(Rev. 173, Issued: 11-22-17, Effective: 11-28-17, Implementation: 11-28-17)

§483.24(a) Based on the comprehensive assessment of a resident and consistent with the resident's needs and choices, the facility must provide the necessary care and services to ensure that a resident's abilities in activities of daily living do not diminish unless circumstances of the individual's clinical condition demonstrate that such diminution was unavoidable. This includes the facility ensuring that:

§483.24(a)(1) A resident is given the appropriate treatment and services to maintain or improve his or her ability to carry out the activities of daily living, including those specified in paragraph (b) of this section...

§483.24(b) Activities of daily living.

The facility must provide care and services in accordance with paragraph (a) for the following activities of daily living:

§483.24(b)(1) Hygiene – bathing, dressing, grooming, and oral care,
§483.24(b)(2) Mobility – transfer and ambulation, including walking,
§483.24(b)(3) Elimination – toileting,
§483.24(b)(4) Dining – eating, including meals and snacks,
§483.24(b)(5) Communication, including

    (i)   **Speech**
    (ii)   **Language**
    (iii)   **Other functional communication systems.**

F677
(Rev. 173, Issued: 11-22-17, Effective: 11-28-17, Implementation: 11-28-17)

§483.24(a)(2) "A resident who is unable to carry out activities of daily living receives the necessary services to maintain good nutrition, grooming, and personal and oral hygiene; and

DEFINITIONS –

"Oral care" refers to the maintenance of a healthy mouth, which includes not only teeth, but the lips, gums, and supporting tissues. This involves not only activities such as brushing of teeth or oral appliances, but also maintenance of oral mucosa.

"Speech, language or other functional communication systems" refers to the resident's ability to effectively communicate requests, needs, opinions, and urgent problems; to express emotion, to listen to others and to participate in social conversation whether in speech, writing, gesture, behavior, or a combination of these (e.g., a communication board of electronic augmentative communication device).

"**Assistance with the bathroom**" refers to the resident's ability to use the toilet room (or commode, bedpan, urinal); transfer on/off the toilet, clean themselves, change absorbent pads or briefs, manage ostomy or catheter, and adjust clothes.

"**Transfer**" refers to resident's ability to move between surfaces – to/from: bed, chair, wheelchair, and standing positions. (Excludes to/from bath/toilet)

GUIDANCE for F676 & F677 (This is abridged form of the guidance; refer to State Operations Manual Appendix PP for the full content of the guidance)

The existence of a clinical diagnosis shall not justify a decline in a resident's ability to perform ADLs unless the resident's clinical picture reflects the normal progression of the disease/condition has resulted in an unavoidable decline in the resident's ability to perform ADLs.

Remarks

Remarks: the two most important statements for these 2 F-tags that you need to be aware of are as follows.

1. CMS has indicated that a resident's decline in their ability to perform their activities of daily living (ADLs) should not just be attributable to the resident's clinical diagnosis. CMS also noted on this GUIDANCE that some of the conditions that may lead to decline in a resident's ability to perform ADLs are:
    a. natural progression of a debilitating disease,
    b. the onset of an acute episode causing physical and/or mental decline, and
    c. a resident and their representative's desire to refuse care, and
    d. depression may also lead to disability and decline
2. Surveyors have the responsibility to determine whether the resident's unavoidable decline occurred after admission, and whether the decline was addressed by the facility staff, whether plan of care was developed to address the resident's decline, and whether the intervention(s) developed in the plan of care were followed by the staff.

F684

(Rev. 173, Issued: 11-22-17, Effective: 11-28-17, Implementation: 11-28-17)
§483.25 Quality of Care

Quality of care is a fundamental principle that applies to all treatment and care provided to facility residents. Based on the comprehensive assessment of a resident, the facility must ensure that residents receive treatment and care in accordance with professional standards of practice, the comprehensive person-centered care plan, and the residents' choices, including but not limited to the following:

INTENT

To ensure facilities identify and provide needed care and services that are resident centered, in accordance with the resident's preferences, goals for care and professional standards of practice that will meet each resident's physical, mental, and psychosocial needs.

DEFINITIONS

"Highest practicable physical, mental, and psychosocial well-being" is defined as the highest possible level of functioning and well-being, limited by the individual's recognized pathology and normal aging process. Highest practicable is determined through the comprehensive resident assessment and by recognizing and competently and thoroughly addressing the physical, mental, or psychosocial needs of the individual.

"Hospice Care" means a comprehensive set of services described in Section 1861(dd)(1) of the Act, identified and coordinated by an interdisciplinary group (IDG) to provide for the physical, psychosocial, spiritual, and emotional needs of a terminally ill patient and/or family members, as delineated in a specific patient plan of care (42 CFR §418.3)

"Palliative care" means patient and family-centered care that optimizes quality of life by anticipating, preventing, and treating suffering. Palliative care throughout the continuum of illness involves addressing physical, intellectual, emotional, social, and spiritual needs and to facilitate patient autonomy, access to information, and choice. (§418.3)

"Terminally ill" means that the individual has a medical prognosis that his or her life expectancy is 6 months or less if the illness runs its normal course. (§418.3)

GUIDANCE (This is an abridged form of the guidance; refer to State Operations Manual Appendix PP for the full content of the guidance)

NOTE: Although Federal requirements dictate the completion of RAI assessments according to certain time frames, standards of good clinical practice dictate that the clinical assessment process is more fluid and should be ongoing. The lack of ongoing clinical assessment and identification of changes in condition, to meet the resident's needs between RAI assessments should be addressed at §483.35 Nursing Services, F726 (competency and skills to identify and address a change in condition), and the relevant outcome tag, such as §483.12 Abuse, §483.24 Quality of Life, §483.25 Quality of Care, and/or §483.40 Behavioral Health.

Remarks

Remarks: I am recommending that as Directors of Nursing, you and your staff should take time to review the GUIDANCE section in the State Operations Manual as it has detailed discussion about the additional items #1 to #9 listed below. You will have further understanding of what the surveyors look for when they come to your facilities for annual surveys and/or compliant surveys. Pay close attention to the statement that tells you that nursing staffs should prioritize your professional practice to identifying what each resident's highest practicable well-being is, in the areas of their physical, mental, and psychosocial health. As the Director of Nursing, your responsibility/ domain is the supervision of the clinical care of the residents. The hierarchy and structure in your facility relating to resident care and services is the administrator then you. You have taken the mantle to ensure that the staffs provide the care and services for the residents to attain and/or maintain the residents' highest practicable physical, mental, and psychosocial well-being.

Below are additional specific topic areas that your nursing staff and other related disciplines must include in their professional practice to meet their responsibilities to provide quality of care and services. Please note that these topic areas listed below are not all inclusive, as there are additional areas not listed that meet the need for Quality of Care.

1. Review of a Resident with Non Pressure-Related Skin Ulcer/Wound
2. Review of a Resident at or Approaching End of Life and/or Receiving Hospice Care and Services
3. Care Plan
4. Resident Care Policies

5. Hospice Care and Services Provided by a Medicare-certified Hospice
6. Coordinated care Plan
7. Physician Services
8. Communication
9. Review of Facility Practices/Written Agreement for Hospice Services

F692
(Rev. 173, Issued: 11-22-17, Effective: 11-28-17, Implementation: 11-28-17)
§483.25(g) Assisted nutrition and hydration.

(Includes naso-gastric and gastrostomy tubes, both percutaneous endoscopic gastrostomy and percutaneous endoscopic jejunostomy, and enteral fluids). Based on a resident's comprehensive assessment, the facility must ensure that a resident-

§483.25(g)(1) Maintain acceptable parameters of nutritional status, such as usual body weight or desirable body weight range and electrolyte balance, unless the resident's clinical condition demonstrates that this is not possible or resident preferences indicate otherwise;

§483.25(g)(2) Is offered sufficient fluid intake to maintain proper hydration and health;

§483.25(g)(3) Is offered a therapeutic diet when there is a nutritional problem and the health care provider orders a therapeutic diet.

INTENT §483.25(g)

The intent of this requirement is that the resident maintains, to the extent possible, acceptable parameters of nutritional and hydration status and that the facility:

- Provides nutritional and hydration care and services to each resident, consistent with the resident's comprehensive assessment;
- Recognizes, evaluates, and addresses the needs of every resident, including but not limited to, the resident at risk or already experiencing impaired nutrition and hydration; and
- Provides a therapeutic diet that takes into account the resident's clinical condition, and preferences, when there is a nutritional indication.

DEFINITIONS §483.25(g)

Definitions are provided to clarify clinical terms related to nutritional status.

"**Acceptable parameters of nutritional status**" refers to factors that reflect that an individual's nutritional status is adequate, relative to his/her overall condition and prognosis, such as weight, food/fluid intake, and pertinent laboratory values.

"**Artificial nutrition and hydration**" are medical treatments and refer to nutrition that is provided through routes other than the usual oral route, typically by placing a tube directly into the stomach, the intestine or a vein.

"**Clinically significant**" refers to effects, results, or consequences that materially affect or are likely to affect an individual's physical, mental, or psychosocial well-being either positively by preventing, stabilizing, or improving a condition or reducing a risk, or negatively by exacerbating, causing, or contributing to a symptom, illness, or decline in status.

"**Dietary supplements**" refers to herbal and alternative products that are not regulated by the Food and Drug Administration and their composition is not standardized. Dietary supplements must be labeled as such and must not be represented for use as a conventional food or as the sole item of a meal or the diet.

"**Health Care Provider**" includes a physician, physician assistant, nurse practitioner, or clinical nurse specialist, or a qualified dietitian or other qualified nutrition professional acting within their state scope of practice and to whom the attending physician has delegated the task. For issue related to delegation to dietitians, refer to §483.60(e)(2)

"**Nutritional status**" includes both nutrition and hydration status.

"**Nutritional Supplements**" refers to products that are used to complement a resident's dietary needs) (e.g., calorie or nutrient dense drinks, total parenteral products, enteral products, and meal replacement products).

"**Therapeutic diet**" refers to a diet ordered by a physician or other delegated provider that is part of the treatment for a disease or clinical condition, to eliminate, decrease, or increase certain substances in the diet (e.g. sodium or potassium), or to provide mechanically altered food when indicated.

"Tube feeding" refers to the delivery of nutrients through a feeding tube directly into the stomach, duodenum, or jejunum. It is also referred to as an enteral feeding.

GUIDANCE §483.25(g) (This is an abridged form of the guidance; refer to the State Operations Manual Appendix PP for the full content of the guidance).

It is important to maintain adequate nutritional status, to the extent possible, to ensure each resident is able to maintain the highest practicable level of well=being. The early identification of residents with, or at risk for, impaired nutrition or hydration status may allow the interdisciplinary team to develop and implement interventions to stabilize or improve nutritional status before complications arise. Body weight and laboratory results can often be stabilized or improved with time, but may not be correctable in some individuals. Intake alone is not the only factor that can affect nutritional status. Resident conditions and co-morbidities may prevent improved nutritional or hydration status, despite improved intake.

Remarks:

Remark - As the nursing staff has responsibility for taking residents weights from admissions through continued residents' stay in the facility, I am also listing below the suggested parameters per the regulation, for identifying and evaluating residents weights. All facilities have their policies and procedures for residents' weights, including the frequency of taking weights for newly admitted residents, and taking weights based on physician orders. Although the frequency is monthly weights for majority of residents whose clinical condition are stable, staffs must pay close attention and follow physician orders for weekly weights or other frequency. Orders for patient/residents' weight must be followed timely as this is important clinical data for the dietitian, as this helps the evaluation and assessment of the residents clinical condition. Both nursing staff and dietitian have to work closely and communicate significant weight loss or weight gain so corrective intervention can be taken by the team. Because F692 is a "Quality of Care" regulation, I recommend that staff spend time reviewing this section in the State Operations Manual as it ccontains additional detailed discussion.

Suggested parameters for evaluating significance of unplanned and undesired weight loss are:

Interval	Significant Loss	Severe Loss
1 month	5%	Greater than 5%
3 months	7.5%	Greater than 7.5%
6 months	10%	Greater than 10%

The following formula determines percentage of weight loss:

% of body weight loss = (usual weight – actual weight) / (usual weight) x 100

F810
(Rev. 173, Issued: 11-22-17, Effective: 11-28-17, Implementation: 11-28-17)
§483.60(g) Assistive devices

The facility must provide special eating equipment and utensils for residents who need them and appropriate assistance to ensure that the resident can use the assistive devices when consuming meals and snacks.

F811
(Rev. 173, Issued 11-22-17, Effective: 11-28-17, Implementation: 11-28-17)
§483.60(h) Paid feeding assistants-

§483.60(h)(1) State approved training course. A facility may use a paid feeding assistant, as defined in § 488.301 of this chapter, if—

> (i)   **A feeding assistant has successfully completed a State-approved training course that meets the requirements of §483.160 before feeding residents; and**
>
> (ii)   **The use of feeding assistants is consistent with State law.**

§483.60(h)(2) Supervision.

(i) A feeding assistant must work under the supervision of a registered nurse (RN) or licensed practical nurse (LPN).

(ii) In an emergency, a feeding assistant must call a supervisory nurse for help.

§483.60(h)(3) Resident selection criteria.

(i) A facility must ensure that a feeding assistant provides dining assistance only for residents who have no complicated feeding problems.

(ii) Complicated feeding problems include, but not limited to, difficulty swallowing, recurrent lung aspirations, and tube or parenteral/IV feedings.

(iii) The facility must base resident selection on the interdisciplinary team's assessment and the resident's latest assessment and plan of care. Appropriateness for this program should be reflected in the comprehensive care plan.

NOTE: Paid feeding assistants must complete a training program with the following minimum content as specified at §483.160.

a. Minimum training course contents. A State-approved training course for paid feeding assistants must include, at minimum, 8 hours of training in the following:
1. Feeding techniques;
2. Assistance with feeding and hydration;
3. Communication and interpersonal skills;
4. Appropriate responses to resident behavior;
5. Safety and emergency procedures, including the Heimlich maneuver;
6. Infection control;
7. Resident rights; and
8. Recognizing changes in residents that are inconsistent with their normal behavior and the importance of reporting those changes to the supervisory nurse.

b. Maintenance of records. A facility must maintain a record of all individuals, used by the facility as feeding assistants, who have successfully completed the training course for paid feeding assistants.

INTENT §483.60(h)(1)-(3) – To ensure that residents are assessed for appropriateness for a feeding assistant program, receive services as per their plan of care, and feeding assistants are trained and supervised. The use of paid feeding assistants is intended to supplement certified nurse aides, not substitute for nurse aides or licensed nursing staff.

DEFINITIONS §483.60(h)(1)-(3)

"Paid feeding assistant" is defined in the regulation at 42 CFR §488.301 as "an individual who meets the requirements specified at 42 CFR §483.60(h)(1)(i) and who is paid by the facility to feed residents, who is used under an arrangement with another agency or organization."

GUIDANCE §483.60(h)(1)-(3)

NOTE: the regulation requires that paid feeding assistants must work under the supervision of an RN or LPN, and they must call the supervisory nurse in case of an emergency. Therefore, a facility that has received a waiver and does not have either an RN or LPN available in the building cannot use paid feeding assistants during those times.

F813
(Rev. 173, Issued: 11-22-17, Effective: 11-28-17, Implementation: 11-28-17)
§483.60(i) Food Safety Requirements

The facility must—

§483.60(i)(3) Have a policy regarding use and storage of foods brought to residents by family and other visitors to ensure safe and sanitary storage, handling, and consumption.

GUIDANCE §483.60(i)(3)

The facility must have a policy regarding food brought to residents by family and other visitors. The policy must also include ensuring facility staff assists that resident in accessing and consuming the food, if the resident is not able to do so on his or her own. The facility also is responsible for storing food brought in by family or visitors in a way that is either separate or easily distinguishable from facility food.

The facility has a responsibility to help family and visitors understand safe food handling practices (such as safe cooling/reheating processes, hot/cold holding temperatures, preventing cross contamination, hand hygiene, etc.). If the facility is assisting family or visitors with reheating or other preparation activities, facility staff must use safe food handling practices.

F947
(Rev. 211; Issued: 02-03-23; Effective: 10-21-22; Implementation: 10-24-22)
§483.95 Training requirements.

Training topics must include but are not limited to—

§483.95(g) Required in-service training for nurse aides.

In-service training must----

§483.95(g)(1) Be sufficient to ensure the continuing competencies of nurse aides, but must be no less than 12 hours per year.

§483.95(g)(2) Include dementia management training and resident abuse prevention training.

§483.95(g)(3) Address areas of weakness as determined in nurse aides' performance reviews and facility assessment at §483.70(e) and may address the special needs of residents as determined by the facility staff.

§483.95(g)(4) For nurse aides providing services to individuals with cognitive impairments, also address the care of the cognitively impaired.

DEFINITIONS

A **"nurse aide"** is defined in §483.5 as any individual providing nursing or nursing-related services to residents in a facility. This term may also include an individual who provides these services through an agency or under a contract with the facility, but is not a licensed health professional, a registered dietitian, or someone who volunteers to provide such services without pay. Nurse aides do not include those individuals who furnish services to residents only as paid feeding assistants as defined in§488.301.

Private duty nurse aides who are not employed or utilized by the facility on a contract, per diem, leased basis, do not come under the nurse aide training provision and therefore are not required to take the training.

Performance Reviews: The process used to evaluate the performance of staff on a periodic basis, which may be annually

GUIDANCE §483.95(g) (This is an abridged form of the guidance; refer to the State Operations Manual Appendix PP for the full content of the guidance)

All facilities must develop, implement and permanently maintain an in-service training program for nurse aides that is appropriate and effective, as determined by nurse aide performance reviews [see §483.35(d)(7)] and the facility assessment as specified at §483.70(e). Changes to the facility's resident population, the facility's physical environment, revisions to the facility's training program.

F948
(Rev. 173, Issued: 11-22-17, Effective: 11-28-17, Implementation: 11-28-17)
§483.95(h) Required training of feeding assistants.

A facility must not use any individual working in the facility as a paid feeding assistant unless that individual has successfully completed a State-approved training program for feeding assistants, as specified in §483.160.

DEFINITION §483.95(h)

Paid feeding assistant is defined in the regulation at 42 CFR §488.301 as "an individual who meets the requirements specified in §483.60(h)(1) of this chapter and who is paid to feed residents by a facility, or who is used under an arrangement with another agency or organization".

Remarks

Remarks - The GUIDANCE section of this F-tag has the requirements for the paid feeding assistants. You as directors of nursing must maintain the training requirements for paid feeding assistants. As stated in the regulation, the training must have the same content as the State -approved training course. The content include feeding techniques, feeding and hydration, interpersonal skills which will help the staff respond appropriately to the residents. The training must also include areas in resident rights, infection control, recognizing changes in residents, safety of residents and training also on performing the Heimlich maneuver. As the one with responsibility for the nursing staff, you must also maintain record of the names of all paid feeding assistants who have undergone the training.

Chapter 7

PRACTICAL TIPS FOR DIRECTORS OF NURSING AND CASE STUDY

As Directors of Nursing, you are in charge of the largest department in the nursing home.. You have the responsibility to ensure that all nursing personnel at all levels have the required competencies to perform their duties successfully in a professional manner, providing quality of care and services and providing quality of life meeting the needs of the residents. You have the responsibility to ensure that the required nursing policies and procedures are in place. You and the Medical Director must work collaboratively to accomplish this task. The Medical Director's role is to supervise the medical care of the residents and your role is to supervise the clinical aspects of the care and supervise your professional nurses and other nursing related personnel either directly or indirectly. It cannot be over-emphasized that directors of nursing and the administrators must work collaboratively as both of you are leaders in the facility.

Residents' nutritional status is an important component of the residents' care planning, and the director of nursing must also be mindful of the residents mealtime experience, particularly for the frail and/or elderly residents, to ensure the residents' nutritional needs are met. Nursing has their role to play in the interdisciplinary process and in helping residents maintain pleasant mealtime experience.

Practical Tips for Director of Nursing:

These are broad administrative, and management tips not clinical tips.

- Ensure that the residents receive Quality of Care and Services, and Quality of Life based on the residents' comprehensive assessments. Residents' meal time experience contributes to the residents' quality of life. Licensed nurses and certified nurse aides as direct caregivers play an important role in ensuring that the care and services the residents receive meet the quality the residents need and deserve.

- Supervision of licensed nurses – registered nurses (RNs), and licensed practical nurses (LPNs) need to make certain that assessments for residents are completed timely upon admission as required; and 48-Hour care plans are initiated by nursing and other appropriate disciplines.

- Work closely with the Medical Director and other team members for developing and updating clinical nursing policies and procedures based the pertinent regulations and Memoranda from CMS, and also upon facility assessments if there is a change in facility resident population and acuity. Also work with physician extenders to ensure clinical care needs of residents/patients are met.

- Work with the Interdisciplinary Team (IDT) and take the lead in ensuring nurse managers and other IDT members update and modify care plans quarterly, annually and whenever there is a change in residents care, particularly when there is a change in condition

- Work with the Dietitian, nurse managers and the Food Service Director/ Manager so that residents' food diets are maintained based on physician orders.

- Have and lead clinical meetings daily (Monday thru Friday) with nurse managers, social service director, rehab (OT, PT), dietitian, and other relevant disciplines and department. Length of meeting could be hour and a half.

- Ensure that nursing staff is aware of the scheduled times residents meal carts are delivered to the unit. Adequate staff should be available when food carts are delivered to the unit, so residents can eat their meals soon thereafter. Enough staff need to be on the unit for mealtimes to render assistance and help with meals. Some facilities practice what they refer to as "all-hands-on-deck", for nurse managers, charge nurses, and the certified nurse aides to be available to help during residents' mealtime.

- Residents' weights must be taken by nursing staff based on facility's policies and procedures, and physician orders, and that the weights are recorded in the medical records; as Dietitian need the data for resident assessment. Nurse Managers, Charge Nurses, certified Nurse Aides/Nursing Assistants to ensure that residents weights are taken as required.

- Ensure the Dietitian is informed of residents who have unusual weight loss or unusual weight gain – this is a "must".

- Ensure line of communication between you and nurse managers, charge nurses and nursing supervisors to keep abreast issues and resolve problems timely.

- Provide support and mentoring for the nursing staff to help them with clinical skills as well as supervisory skills if and when needed.

- Hiring of nursing staff at all levels and ensure that there is adequate staff to provide care and that staff receive their required mandatory in-services and competencies. Annual employee performance evaluations to be done timely so staff can get feedback on their performance.

- Work very closely with the administrator and keep line of communication open, and report to him/her any unusual incidents, situations, complaints or grievances for timely resolutions. Also report unusual incidents to the appropriate state agency in a timely manner as required by the state law or regulation.

- Engage your staff in survey preparation for annual certification survey, so nursing department is in regulatory compliance and always survey ready 365 days a year.

- Participate in clinical rounds at minimum weekly.

- Be an integral member of the facility's Quality Assurance Performance Improvement (QAPI) Program and determine which nursing data should be reported at committee meetings.

- Work with social service director and MDS coordinator to review schedules for IDT meetings and care plan updates.

- Have biweekly meetings with nurse managers, and monthly meetings with all nursing staff

For the case study below, you can work on it independently or work collaboratively with members of your team.

CASE STUDY

DISCLAIMER: This case study is fictional – fictional names of skilled nursing facilities and/or nursing homes, fictional situations and stories. The names, characters and incidents portrayed in the case studies are fictional, and no identification with persons (living or dead) and with places or with products should be assumed or inferred.

CASE STUDY-

On a Wednesday afternoon during mealtime for lunch, the nurse manager was called to the dining room by the certified nurse aide. The nurse aide informed the nurse manager that one of the residents, said that she could not eat the fish she had on her plate. She told the nurse aide: "I can't eat this. Don't you know I don't like fish? Fish usually makes me want to throw up and it sometimes gives me rash. I told the nurse that spoke to me a couple days ago when she was asking me questions after I was admitted, I told her that I don't like fish, and she said that she would write it down on my record."

The nurse manager came to the dining room and asked the resident what the problem was. Nurse Manager said to the resident: "they told me you don't want to eat this nice fish they serve you today." The resident: "Yes, I am not even sure why you are asking, because you people should know that I don't eat fish." The nurse manager responded "I am sorry about that, we will let the kitchen know and we will send you a substitute meal. Let's see what they have in the kitchen. Do you want hamburger and fries, or do you want sandwich and salad?. Again, I apologize."

The nurse manager spoke to the Food Service Supervisor promptly to resolve the issue and the resident did receive her substitute tray for lunch in a relatively timely manner.

This issue was brought to the Director of Nursing's (DON's) attention, and the DON called an impromptu meeting with the nurse managers to address the issue. The DON asked that the nurse manager access the resident's chart in the computer. They reviewed the documentation on the resident's admission assessment performed by the registered nurse. The documentation revealed that the admission assessment was performed by a newly hired nurse on the unit.

Identify some of the issues and solutions to prevent something like this from not happening again. Utilizing some of the questions below how will you prevent this issue and similar issues so you do not have the same or similar matters happen in the future?

EXERCISES TO DO

For Directors of Nursing

As Director of Nursing, how will you handle this situation, or similar situations to prevent a recurrence?

The most important hint or rule is "Do not blame the people (staff); look at your systems.

A. How will you set up your root cause analysis to ensure that this situation of diet likes and dislikes and/or allergies are captured and documented?

B. What do you need to do about orientation for new nurses to the facility?

C. Reviewing your policies and procedures for clinical assessments of newly admitted residents, does your policy and procedure include "resident meal time", and meeting the nutritional needs of residents? If not, how do you communicate this important aspect of care to the nursing staff as well as to the kitchen?

D. What do you need to have on your QAPI Report for the Root Cause Analysis and what measures need to be initiated for the Interdisciplinary Team (IDT) regarding care planning?

E. Does the Dietitian and/or the Food Service Department have responsibility to bear on this issue of knowing likes and dislikes of newly admitted residents on a timely manner?

F. What other areas do you think need to be pursued, relative to this matter to ensure the residents have pleasant meal time experience?

The next section is on Dietitians, and the specific regulations for Dietitians' duties, Tips for Dietitians, and Exercises for the case study for the Dietitians.

Chapter 8

DIETITIANS ROLE AND F-TAG FOCUS

Questions for Dietitians and F-Tags

The Dietitian is one of the most if not the most important discipline in the Interdisciplinary Team (IDT) when it comes to ensuring that residents in Skilled Nursing Facilities and Nursing Homes meet their nutritional needs and maintains their nutritional status. Majority of the residents who live in the nursing homes are elderly some of whom are frail and others with comorbidities, requiring very special needs. With Resident Rights, and person-centered care there is focus on individualized care and residents preferences, likes, dislikes and food choices.

Resident rights, resident self-determination, diagnoses, person-centered care, individualized care, food likes, dislikes, cultural and ethnic food needs, religious requirements, and allergies etc. are all incorporated into the dietitian's decision making process in meeting the nutritional needs of the residents. The dietitians must maintain the required competencies, skills set, professional standards, and knowledge of the long term care regulations F-tags in order to assess and determine the residents' nutritional status and meet their needs. Thus dietitian must also help to make sure that the residents attain or maintain their highest practicable physical, mental and psychosocial well-being..

Below are questions for the dietitians. Utilize these for your self-assessment towards your duties and responsibilities. Review and answer the questions on the space between questions as you desire.

Questions For Dietitians:

1. How much of the Food and Nutrition Services F-tags of the Federal Long Term Care Regulations do you know and feel comfortable with? The idea is for you to have a comfort level with what you should know.

2. How well do you communicate and interact with the Director of Nursing and Nurse Managers for timely developing and updating of residents care plans?

3. How well do you follow up with the attending physician and nursing staff to ensure that there is diet order for residents newly admitted to the facility, and for those residents that may have had a change in condition?

4. If your State regulations allow the physician to delegate diet orders to you as the Dietitian, how well do you and the physician coordinate and communicate to ensure that the system works well?

5. How do you see your role and participation in daily clinical meetings and in the Interdisciplinary Care Plan Meetings?

6. If residents' weights are not taken by nursing staff timely, and care plans are not developed and/or updated timely how effectively do you address those situations?

7. In developing cycle menus for the residents, who or which participants are part of the team that gives input to help with suggestions of menu items, and why did you include them in the team?

8. Do your cycle menus reflect seasonal changes in foods such as fruits and vegetables to offer residents a variety?

9. How well do you work with the Director of Nursing and the Food Service Director/ Manager, to accomplish quality of care, quality of life for residents health and well-being?

10. Do you participate in the facility's QAPI program, and what routine reporting of data do you contribute to the reporting cycle?

F-Tags for Dietitians
F800
(Rev. 173, Issued: 11-22-17, Effective: 11-28-17, Implementation: 11-28-17)
§483.60 Food and nutrition services

The facility must provide each resident with a nourishing, palatable, well-balanced diet that meets his or her daily nutritional and special dietary needs, taking into consideration the preferences of each resident.

INTENT §483.60 – To ensure that facility staff support the nutritional well-being of the residents while respecting an individual's right to make choices about his or her diet.

GUIDANCE §483.60

This requirement expects that there is ongoing communication and coordination among and between staff within all departments to ensure that the resident assessment, care plan and actual food and nutrition services meet each resident's daily nutritional and dietary needs and choices.

While it may be challenging to meet every resident's individual preferences, incorporating a resident's preferences and dietary needs will ensure residents are offered meaningful choices in meals/diets that are nutritionally adequate and satisfying to the individual. Reasonable efforts to accommodate these choices and preferences must be addressed by facility staff.

F801
(Rev. 207; Issued 09-30-22; Effective: 09-30-22; Implementation: 10-01-22)
§483.60(a) Staffing

The facility must employ sufficient staff with the appropriate competencies and skills sets to carry out the functions of the food and nutrition service, taking into consideration resident assessments, individual plans of care and the number, acuity and diagnoses of the facility's resident population in accordance with the facility assessment required at §483.70(e)

This includes:

§483.60(a)(1) A qualified dietitian or other clinically qualified nutrition professional either full-time, part-time, or on a consultant basis. A qualified dietitian or other clinically qualified nutrition professional is one who—

- (i) **Holds a bachelor's or higher degree granted by a regionally accredited college or university in the United States (or an equivalent foreign degree) with completion of the academic requirements of a program in nutrition or dietetics accredited by an appropriate national accreditation organization recognized for this purpose.**
- (ii) **Has completed at least 900 hours of supervised dietetics practice under the supervision of a registered dietitian or nutrition professional.**
- (iii) **Is licensed or certified as a dietitian or nutritional professional by the State in which the services are performed. In a State that does not provide for licensure or certification, the individual will be deemed to have met this requirement if he or she is recognized as a "registered dietitian" by**

the Commission on Dietetic Registration or its successor organization, or meets the requirements of paragraphs (a)(1)(i) and (ii) of this section.

(iv) For dietitian hired or contracted with prior to November 28, 2016, meets these requirements no later than 5 years after November 28, 2016 or as required by state law.

§483.60(a)(2) If a qualified dietitian or other clinically qualified nutrition professional is not employed full-time, the facility must designate a person to serve as the director of food and nutrition services—

(i) The director of food and nutrition services must at a minimum meet one of the following qualifications—

A. A certified dietary manager; or
B. A certified food service manager; or
C. Has similar national certification for food service management and safety from a national certifying body; or
D. Has an associate's or higher degree in food service management or in hospitality, if the course study includes food service or restaurant management, from an accredited institution of higher learning; or
E. Has 2 or more years of experience in the position of director of food and nutrition services in a nursing facility setting and has completed a course of study in food safety and management, by no later than October 1, 2023, that includes topics integral to managing dietary operations including, but not limited to, foodborne illness, sanitation procedures, and food purchasing/receiving; and

(ii) In States that have established standards for food service managers or dietary managers, meets State requirements for food service managers or dietary managers, and

(iii) Receives frequently scheduled consultations from a qualified dietitian or other clinically qualified nutrition professional.

INTENT §483.60 (a)(1)-(2) – To ensure there is sufficient and qualified staff with the appropriate competencies and skill sets to carry out food and nutrition services.

DEFINITIONS §483.60(a)(1)-(2)

"Full-time" means working 35 hours or more a week

"Part-time" employees typically work fewer hours in a day or during a work week than full-time employees. The U.S. Department of Labor, Bureau of Statistics uses a definition of 34 or fewer hours a week as part-time work. Part-time workers may also be those who only work during certain parts of the year.

"Consultant" means an individual who gives professional advice or services. They are generally not direct employees of the facility and may work either full or part-time.

GUIDANCE §483.60(a)(1)-(2)

Cite F801 for concerns regarding the qualifications of the dietitian, other clinical nutrition professionals, or the food services director. For concerns regarding support personnel refer to F802, Sufficient Dietary support Personnel.

In addition, cite F801 if staff, specifically the qualified dietitian or other clinically qualified nutrition professional did not carry out the functions of the food and nutrition services. While these functions may be defined by facility management, at a minimum they should include, but are not limited to:

- Assessing the nutritional needs of residents;
- Developing and evaluating regular and therapeutic diets, including texture of foods and liquids, to meet the specialized need of residents;
- Developing and implementing person centered education programs involving food and nutrition services for all facility staff;
- Overseeing the budget and purchasing of food and supplies, and food preparation, service and storage; and,
- Participating in the quality assurance and performance (QAPI), as described in §483.75, when food and nutrition services are involved.

The qualified dietitian or other clinically qualified nutrition professional can decide to oversee and delegate some of the activities listed above to the director of food and nutrition services.

F803
(Rev. 173, Issued: 11-22-17, Effective: 11-28-17, Implementation: 11-28-17)
§483.60(c) Menus and nutritional adequacy.
Menus must—
§483.60(c)(1) "Meet the nutritional needs of residents in accordance with established national guidelines;

§483.60(c)(2) Be prepared in advance;

§483.60(c)(3) Be followed

§483.60(c)(4) Reflect, based on a facility's reasonable efforts, the religious, cultural and ethnic needs of the resident population, as well as input received from residents and resident groups;

§483.60(c)(5) Be updated periodically;

§483.60(c)(6) Be reviewed by the facility's dietitian or other clinically qualified nutrition professional for nutritional adequacy; and

§483.60(c)(7) Nothing in this paragraph should be construed to limit the resident's right to make personal dietary choices.

INTENT §483.60(c)(1)-(7) – To assure that menus are developed and prepared to meet resident choices including their nutritional, religious, cultural, and ethnic needs while using established national guidelines.

DEFINITIONS §483.60(c)(1)-(7)

"Reasonable effort" means assessing individual resident needs and preferences and demonstrating actions to meet those needs and preferences, including reviewing availability of procurement sources of such food items, identifying preparation methods and approaches, and determining whether purchasing and serving such items can occur.

"Periodically" means that a facility should update its menus to accommodate their changing resident population or resident needs as determined by their facility assessment. See F838. This includes ethnic, cultural, or religious factors that may potentially affect the care provided by the facility, including, but not limited to, activities and food and nutrition services.

GUIDANCE §483.60(c)(1-7)

The facility must make reasonable efforts to provide food that is appetizing to and culturally appropriate for residents. This means learning the resident's needs and preferences and responding to them. For residents with dementia or other barriers or challenges to expressing their preferences, facility staff should document the steps taken to learn what those preferences are.

It is not required that there be individualized menus for all residents; however, alternatives aligned with individual needs and preferences should be available if the primary menu or immediate selections for a particular meal are not to a resident's liking. Facilities must reasonable and good faith efforts to develop a menu based on resident request and resident groups' feedback.

F805
(Rev. 173, Issued: 11-22-17, Effective: 11-28-17, Implementation: 11-28-17)
§483.60(d) Food and drink
Each resident receives and the facility provides—
§483.60(d)(3) Food prepared in a form designed to meet individual needs.

F806
(Rev. 173, Issued: 11-22-17, Effective: 11-28-17, Implementation: 11-28-17)
§483.60(d) Food and drink
Each resident receives and the facility provides—
§483.60(d)(4) Food that accommodates resident allergies, intolerances, and preferences;
§483.60(d)(5) Appealing options of similar nutritive value to residents who choose not to eat food that is initially served or who request a different meal choice; and

GUIDANCE §483.60(d)(4)-(5)
Facilities should be aware of each resident's allergies, intolerances, and preferences, and provide an appropriate alternative. A food substitute should be consistent with the usual and/or ordinary food items provided by the facility. For example, the facility may, instead of grapefruit juice, substitute another citrus juice or vitamin C rich juice the resident likes.

F807
(Rev. 173, Issued: 11-22-17, Effective: 11-28-17, Implementation: 11.28-17)
§483.60(d) Food and drink
Each resident receives and the facility provides—
§483.60(d)(6) Drinks, including water and other liquids consistent with resident needs and preferences and sufficient to maintain resident hydration.

GUIDANCE §483.60(d)(6)

Proper hydration alone is a critical aspect of nutrition among nursing home residents. Individuals who do not receive adequate fluids are more susceptible to urinary tract infections, pneumonia, decubitus ulcers, skin infections, confusion and disorientation.

F808
(Rev. 173, Issued: 11-22-17, Effective: 11-28-17, Implementation: 11-28-17)
§483.60(e) Therapeutic Diets
$483.60(e)(1) Therapeutic diets must be prescribed by the attending physician.
§483.60(e)(2) The attending physician may delegate to a registered or licensed dietitian the task of prescribing a resident's diet, including a therapeutic diet, to the extent allowed by State law.

INTENT §483.60(e)(1)-(2) – To assure that residents receive and consume foods in the appropriate form and/or the appropriate nutritive content as prescribed by a physician, and/or assessed by the interdisciplinary team to support the resident's treatment, plan of care, in accordance with his her goals and preferences.

GUIDANCE §483.60(e)(1)-(2)

If the resident's attending physician delegates this task he or she must supervise the dietitian and remains responsible for the resident's care even if the task is delegated. The physician would be able to modify a diet order with a subsequent order, if necessary.

F809
(Rev. 173, Issued: 11-22-17, Effective: 11-28-17, Implementation: 11-28-17)
§483.60(f) Frequency of Meals

§483.60(f)(1) Each resident must receive and the facility must provide at least three meals daily, at regular times comparable to normal mealtimes in the community or in accordance with resident needs, preferences, requests, and plan of care.

§483.60(f)(2) There must be no more than 14 hours between a substantial evening meal and breakfast the following day, except when a nourishing snack is served at bedtime, up to 16 hours may elapse between a substantial evening meal and breakfast the following day if a resident group agrees to this meal span.

§483.60(f)(3) Suitable, nourishing, alternative meals and snacks must be provided to residents who want to eat at non-traditional times or outside of the scheduled meal service times, consistent with the resident plan of care.

DEFINITIONS §483.60(f)(1)-(3)

A **"Nourishing snack"** "means items from the basic food groups, either singly or in combination with each other.

"Suitable and nourishing alternative meals and snacks" means that when an alternate meal or snack is provided, it is of similar nutritive value as the meal or snack offered at the normally scheduled time and consistent with the resident plan of care.

Remarks

Remarks: Based on what the surveyors look for when they come to your facility, they will observe the snacks you provide for the residents. They will look for: (1) whether the snacks are of nutritive value, (2) whether the snacks given to the residents are determined based on the residents assessments, (3) whether the snacks are documented in the residents plans of care or medical records, (4), whether the plans of care contain the types of snacks the resident should receive, and (5) whether the staff knows the times that the snacks should be served their snacks.

If and when managers are monitoring facility practice for compliance of the regulations, their observations should confirm whether snacks provided meet the residents' plan of care. There some situations when residents are served the snacks, but staff are not available to assist some of the residents in consuming their snacks.

Dietitians, you may want to continue to work with the food service manager to ensure that suitable and nourishing alternative meals are available and must be provided for those residents who may choose to eat their meals at different times as opposed to the regular scheduled facility's mealtime. The facility should make allowance for those residents to eat at the time they may prefer. The surveyors may ask questions of the residents about their preferences for meals and snacks.

F813
(Rev. 173, Issued: 11-22-17, Effective: 11-28-17, Implementation: 11-28-17)
§483.60(i) Food Safety Requirements

The facility must—
§483.60(i)(3) Have a policy regarding use and storage of foods brought to residents by family and other visitors to ensure safe and sanitary storage, handling, and consumption.

GUIDANCE §483.60(i)(3)

The facility must have a policy regarding food brought to residents by family and other visitors. The policy must also include ensuring facility staff assists the resident in accessing and consuming the food, if the resident is not able to do so on his or her own. The facility also is responsible for storing food brought in by family or visitors in a way that is either separate or easily distinguishable from facility food.

"The facility has a responsibility to help family and visitors understand safe food handling practices (such as safe cooling/reheating processes, hot/cold holding temperatures, preventing cross contamination, hand hygiene, etc.). If the facility is assisting family or visitors with reheating or other preparation activities, facility staff must use safe food handling practices.

The next section below addresses two areas of the regulations which are usually described as the fundamentals of **Quality of Life –F675 and Quality of Care - F684.** All disciplines and departments in the nursing homes, and the long term care community must embrace these two (2) F-tags regulations, to understand their importance and understand the role they play in the residents life in the nursing home setting.. These F-tags give us the road map to what the expectations are for the quality of the care and services the residents must receive and deserve.

F675
(Rev. 211: Issued: 02-03-23; Effective: 10-21-22; Implementation: 10-24-22)
§483.24 Quality of Life

Quality of life is a fundamental principle that applies to all care and services provided to facility residents. Each resident must receive and the facility must provide the necessary care and services to attain or maintain the highest practicable physical, mental, and psychosocial well-being, consistent with the resident's comprehensive assessment and plan of care.

INTENT

The intent of this requirement is to specify the facility's responsibility to create and sustain an environment that humanizes and individualizes each resident's quality of life by:

- Ensuring all staff, across all shifts and departments, understand the principles of quality of life, and honor and support these principles for each resident; and
- Ensuring that the care and services provided are person-centered, and honor and support each resident's preferences, choices, values and beliefs.

DEFINITIONS §483.24

"Person Centered Care" – For the purposes of this subpart, person-centered care means to focus on the resident as the locus of control and support the resident in making their own choices and having control over their daily lives. (Definitions - §483.5)

"Pervasive" - For the purposes of this guidance, pervasive means spread through or embedded within every part of something.

"Quality of Life" refers to an individual's "sense of well-being, level of satisfaction with life and feeling of self-worth and self-esteem. For nursing home residents, this includes a basic sense of satisfaction with oneself, the environment, the care received, the accomplishments of desired goals, and control over one's life." Adapted from the 1986 Institute of Medicine (IOM) published report "Improving the Quality of Care in Nursing Homes." Located at: https://www.ncbi.nlm.nih.gov/books/NBK217548/#ddd00037

GUIDANCE §483.24 (This is an abridged form of the guidance for F675; refer to the State Operations Manual Appendix PP for the full content of the guidance).

Noncompliance at F675 identifies outcomes which rise to the level of immediate jeopardy and reflect an environment of pervasive disregard for the quality of life of the facility's residents. This can include the cumulative effect of noncompliance as other regulatory tags on one or more residents. To cite noncompliance at F675, the survey team must have evidence that outcomes at other regulatory tags demonstrate a pervasive disregard for the principles of quality of life.

Facilities must create and sustain an environment that humanizes and promotes each resident's well-being, and feeling of self-worth and self-esteem. This requires nursing home leadership to establish a culture that treats each resident with respect and dignity as an individual, and addresses, supports and/or enhances his/her feelings of self-worth including personal control over choices, such as mealtimes, activities, clothing, and bedtime; privacy during visits, and treatments; and opportunities to engage in religious, political, civic, recreational or other social activities.

F684
(Rev. 173, Issued: 11-22-17, Effective: 11-28-17, Implementation: 11-28-17)
§483.25 Quality of care

Quality of care is a fundamental principle that applies to all treatment and care provided to facility residents. Based on the comprehensive assessment of a resident, the facility must ensure that residents receive treatment and care in accordance with professional standards of practice, the comprehensive person-centered care plan, and the residents' choices, including but not limited to the following:

INTENT

To ensure facilities identify and provide needed care and services that are resident centered, in accordance with the resident's preferences, goals for care and professional standards of practice that will meet each resident's physical, mental, and psychosocial needs.

DEFINITIONS

"Highest practicable physical, mental, and psychosocial well-being" is defined as the highest possible level of functioning and well-being, limited by the individual's recognized pathology and normal aging process. Highest practicable is determined through the comprehensive resident assessment and by recognizing and competently and thoroughly addressing the physical, mental or psychosocial needs of the individual.

"Hospice Care" means a comprehensive set of services described in Section 1861 (dd)(1) of the Act, identified and coordinated by an interdisciplinary group (IDG) to provide for the physical, psychosocial, spiritual, and emotional needs of a terminally ill patient and/or family members, as delineated in a specific patient plan of care. (42 CFR §418.3)

"Palliative care" means patient and family-centered care that optimizes quality of life by anticipating, preventing, and treating suffering. Palliative care throughout the continuum of illness involves addressing physical, intellectual, emotional, social, and spiritual needs and to facilitate patient autonomy, access to information, and choice. (§418.3)

"**Terminally ill**" means that the individual has a medical prognosis that his or her life expectancy is 6 months or less if the illness runs its normal course. (§418.3)

GUIDANCE (This is an abridged form of the guidance for F684; refer to the State Operations Manual for Appendix PP for the full content of the guidance)

Nursing homes must place priority on identifying what each resident's highest practicable well-being is in each of the areas of physical, mental and psychosocial health. Each resident's care plan must reflect person-centered care, and include resident choices, preferences, goals, concerns/needs, and describe the services and care that is to be furnished to attain or maintain, or improve the resident's highest practicable physical, mental and psychosocial well-being. For concerns related to the resident's comprehensive care plan, see F656, §483.21(b) Comprehensive Care Plans.

F692
(Rev. 173, Issued 11-22-17, Effective: 11-28-17, Implementation: 11-28-17)
§483.25(g) Assisted nutrition and hydration.

(Includes naso-gastric and gastrostomy tubes, both percutaneous endoscopic gastrostomy and percutaneous endoscopic jejunostomy, and enteral fluids). Based on a resident's comprehensive assessment, the facility must ensure that a resident—

§483.25(g)(1) Maintains acceptable parameters of nutritional status, such as usual body weight or desirable body weight range and electrolyte balance, unless the resident's clinical condition demonstrates that that this is not possible or resident preferences indicate otherwise;

§483.25(g)(2) Is offered sufficient fluids intake to maintain proper hydration and health;

§483.25(g)(3) Is offered a therapeutic diet when there is a nutritional problem and the health care provider orders a therapeutic diet.

INTENT §483.25(g)

The intent of this requirement is that the resident maintains, to the extent possible, acceptable parameters of nutritional and hydration status and that the facility:

- Provides nutritional and hydration care and services to each resident, consistent with the resident's comprehensive assessment;

- Recognizes, evaluates, and addresses the needs of every resident, including but not limited to, the resident at risk or already experiencing impaired nutrition and hydration; and
- Provides a therapeutic diet that takes into account the resident's clinical condition, and preferences, when there is a nutritional indication.

DEFINITIONS §483.25(g)

Definitions are provided to clarify clinical terms related to nutritional status.

"Acceptable parameters of nutritional status" refers to factors that reflect that an individual's nutritional status is adequate, relative to his/her overall condition and prognosis, such as weight, food/fluid intake, and pertinent laboratory values.

"Artificial nutrition and hydration" are medical treatments and refer to nutrition that is provided through routes other than the usual oral route, typically by placing a tube directly into the stomach, the intestine or a vein.

"Clinically significant" refers to effects, results, or consequences that materially affect or are likely to affect an individual's physical, mental, or psychosocial well-being either positively by preventing, stabilizing, or improving a condition or reducing a risk, or negatively by exacerbating, causing, or contributing to a symptom, illness, or decline in status.

"Dietary supplements" refers to a herbal and alternative products that are not regulated by the Food and Drug Administration and their composition is not standardized. Dietary supplements must be labeled as such and must not be represented for use as a conventional food or as the sole item of a meal or the diet.

"Health Care Provider" includes a physician, physician assistant, nurse practitioner, or clinical nurse specialist, or a qualified dietitian or other qualified nutrition professional acting within their state scope of practice and to whom the attending physician has delegated the task. For issues related to delegation to dietitians, refer to §483.60(e)(2), F808

"Nutritional status" includes both nutrition and hydration status.

"Nutritional Supplements" refers to products that are used to complement a resident's dietary needs (e.g. calorie or nutrient dense drinks, total parenteral products, enteral products, and meal replacement products).

"Therapeutic diet" refers to a diet ordered by a physician or other delegated provider that is part of the treatment for a disease or clinical condition, to eliminate, decrease, or increase certain substances in the diet (e.g., sodium or potassium) or to provide mechanically altered food when indicated.

"Tube feeding" refers to the delivery of nutrients through a feeding tube directly into the stomach, duodenum, or jejunum. It is also referred to as an enteral feeding.

GUIFDANCE §483.25(g) (This is an abridged form of the guidance; refer to the State Operations Manual Appendix PP for the full content of the guidance)

It is important to maintain adequate nutritional status, to the extent possible, to ensure each resident is able to maintain the highest practicable level of well-being. The early identification of residents with, or at risk for, impaired nutrition or hydration status may allow the interdisciplinary team to develop and implement interventions to stabilize or improve nutritional status before complications arise. Body weight and laboratory results can often be stabilized or improved with time, but may not be correctable in some individuals. Intake alone is not the only factor that can affect nutritional status. Resident conditions and co-morbidities may prevent improved nutritional or hydration status, despite improved intake.

Many factors can influence weight and nutritional status as one ages. The body may not absorb or use nutrients as effectively, there may be changes in the ability to take food, or there may be a decreased sensation for thirst or hunger. The resident's medical condition cam also affect how well they maintain weight, such as changes in muscle mass, cognitive status, nearing end of life, or a disease process, such as kidney disease or congestive heart failure, which may cause the resident to retain fluids in the body. While impaired nutritional status is not necessarily expected as one ages, there could be times where efforts to maintain good nutrition may pose extra challenges.

See the suggested parameters for evaluating unplanned and undesired weight loss

"Suggested parameters for evaluating significance of unplanned and undesired weight loss are:"

Interval	Significant Loss	Severe Loss
1 month	5%	Greater than 5%
3 months	7.5%	Greater than 7.5%
6 months	10%	Greater than 10%

Remark

Remarks – Below are some additional areas of focus for the dietitian and other members of the IDT.

There must be collaboration between the dietitian and nursing for the residents weights, particularly the regularity of when residents weights are taken by nursing and the reporting of residents weight. The significance of this routine is for nursing staff to embrace the facility policy and procedure on taking residents weight, and conduct follow up procedure when there is weight loss and/or weight gain. Staffs must be familiar with the table above that denotes the parameters for unplanned significant and/or severe weight loss or gain, so the dietitian can assess residents. The dietitian will complete assessment of residents with significant or severe weight loss to identify potential reason for the weight loss and collaborate with the resident's attending physician, and director of nursing to get possible clinical interventions for any impending clinical or medical problems.

The goal is for the systems within your facilities and your staffs to enable the residents to live up to and maintain and/or improve in their highest practicable physical, mental, and psychosocial well-being. The GUIDANCE also gives you an insight into some of the negative outcomes of the failure to identify residents at risk for compromised nutrition and hydration. Such negative outcome includes increased risk of mortality, increased risk of impairment of anticipated healing, decline in function and issues with fluid and electrolyte imbalance.

Part of the admission process is for nursing, the dietitian and other disciplines to do comprehensive assessment of the residents' needs and clinical status to develop the residents' plans of care. It is also stressed in the guidance for the interdisciplinary team, to continue to (1) assess the residents' needs; (2) reassess the residents' needs; (3) initiate, review and update plans of care and interventions as appropriate (4) continue to monitor the outcomes of interventions and the plans of care to ensure the interventions are working otherwise to make changes to the interventions; (5) document as you go through this process of intervention, plans of care, and outcomes., as documentation is very important.

Chapter 9

PRACTICAL REGULATORY COMPLIANCE TIPS FOR DIETITIANS AND CASE STUDY

Practical Tips – administrative; non-clinical

- **Understand your paramount role in the Interdisciplinary Team (IDT),**
    - As the dietitian you need to take the lead in making certain that residents' nutritional needs are met.
    - Participate in the review and updating of policies and procedures relating to nutritional needs and status of residents, residents mealtime and dining experience.

- **Always remember about person-centered care concept and focus**
    - Each resident is an individual
    - Person-centered care must be the goal.
    - If residents preferences and choices are not reflected in the admission assessment, ask the question and make sure you have it on record and communicate to nursing

- **Be cognizant of residents' frailty and clinical vulnerabilities and co-morbidities**
    - High percentage of the residents are very elderly and frail
    - Complete accurate clinical assessments timely to (a) help these residents maintain and/or improve their health goals, (b) to help them maintain or improve their physical, mental and psychosocial well-being.

- **It is essential to work collaboratively with:**
    - the Director of Nursing,
    - Nurse Managers, Charge Nurses, Nursing Supervisors
    - Rehab Directors and managers as needed

- o Food Service Director/Manager for resident care and pleasant meal time experience.
- o Food Service Supervisors, and of course
- o The Administrator

- **Conduct all clinical assessments accurately, and timely** - admission, comprehensive, quarterly and annually;
  - o Also assessments must be completed if there is change in condition for any resident.

- **Participate in daily clinical meetings to:**
  - o Review new admissions nutritional status with the team
  - o Report and address nutrition related clinical physician orders with the team,
  - o Report any resident weight issues particularly residents unexpected weight loss
  - o Address interventions and possible plans of care..

- **Bring to attention of the team other additional issues with plans of care such as:**
  - o Lack of nutrition plan of care by a discipline to address nutritional issues
  - o Lack of updating or modifying of plan of care by a discipline as required

- **Participate and be an integral part of the IDT meetings.** Must always have a presence in IDT meetings.

- **Nursing staff taking and recording of residents weights: are essential**
  - o Report to the Director of Nursing when residents weights are not taken
  - o .Communicate also to Nurse Managers and Nursing Supervisors alternatively when residents weights not taken
  - o Communicate to Director of Nursing and the residents' attending physicians residents with weight loss and weight gains outside of the CMS parameters

- **Develop and design cycle menus for residents and for the facility.** Seek input from residents and resident groups when developing the menu and the cycle time frame.

- **Follow job descriptions and responsibilities.**

- **Be part of QAPI and establish reporting of data and issues as required by the QAPI Director/Manager/Coordinator.**

- **Ensure that your license and certificate are current, and maintain competencies and continuing education as required.**

CASE STUDY

DISCLAIMER: This case study is fictional – fictional names of skilled nursing facilities and/or nursing homes, fictional situations and fictional stories. The names, characters and incidents portrayed in the case studies are fictional, and no identification with persons (living or dead) and with places or with products should be assumed or inferred.

CASE STUDY

The Dietitian at ABC Skilled Nursing Facility did not receive the monthly weights for five (5) residents on one of the units. All other units at the facility had the monthly weights taken and recorded in the residents' charts/medical records. It so happened, the dietitian and the nurse manager at the unit where the five weights were not taken, for some reason, do not have a good working relationship with each other. So communication between the Dietitian and the Nurse Manager does not usually go well.

The nurse aide who was assigned to take care of the resident on a particular day observed that the resident did not eat her breakfast and her lunch well as she used to. The nurse aide asked the resident, "I noticed you did not eat all your food as you used to, is everything okay? Are you feeling okay?" Resident said "Oh yes, everything is okay, I am fine." The nurse aide however informed the unit manager of her observation concerning the resident; that the resident did not eat her meals like she used to, and that the resident said that everything was okay.

The nurse manager went in to talk to the resident to find out if she was really okay. The nurse manager decided to assess the resident and she took the resident's vital signs, Vital signs were a little off, so the nurse manager went to review the resident's chart. Nurse Manager realized that the patient's weight that should have been taken three days prior was not done, as it was not recorded in the chart. The nurse manager asked some additional questions as part of her assessment, and the resident told the nurse manager that she really was not feeling like eating much lately.

The nurse manager then asked the resident whether she mind being weighed so they could check her out to make sure everything was okay, or if there was something else going on that she might not be aware of. The resident was weighed, and the resident had lost more than five pounds (<5lbs) for that month. Based on the facility policy and procedure the resident was weighed again to validate the weight loss. The re-weigh validated the 5lb weight loss for the month. This was reported to the DON. The nurse manager then informed the DON what had happened and she also told the DON that no one reported to her that the resident had not been weighed for the month. The nurse manager then informed the resident's attending physician, so appropriate action can be taken.

The DON then called a meeting with the dietitian and the nurse manager to find out why the lack of communication that resulted in the nurse manager and the dietitian not aware that the resident's weight was not taken as scheduled. The DON asked the dietitian to takes steps to ensure that this does not happen again.

Exercises for Dietitians To Do

A. As the Dietitian, what is the first action that you need to take to correct this situation immediately?

B. Is this an issue for all members of the Interdisciplinary Team (IDT) to address, if it is, what should be the discussion for corrective measures, if not which members of the IDT should be in discussion to come up with corrective measures, and why?

C. What system needs to be put in place and what follow up measures need to be in place?

D. What should be the involvement of the Director of Nursing in this matter?

E. What do you see as the need for Staff Development, for staff competencies, and for professional communication?

F. Should this be reported to QAPI? Why or why not?

G. Any other additional measures you want to articulate?

PART

5

Chapter 10

FOOD SERVICE DIRECTOR/MANAGER ROLE AND F-TAG FOCUS

Questions for Food Service Director/Manager and F-Tags Focus

As administrator at my facilities, I have always maintained a very good working relationship with my Food and Nutrition Services Department - the department head, the supervisors and the staff. I did this for a few important reasons: Due to my passion for patient/resident care and because I have directly participated and helped with the monitoring for compliance as well as monitoring for resident quality of life. I had developed monitoring tools for resident meal time and dining experience. I cannot overemphasize that residents must maintain their nutritional status, their quality of life, quality of care and services while in the SNFs/Nursing Homes. The Food Service Director/Manager also has vital role to play in Quality of Care and Quality of Life for the residents.

The questions below are for your self-assessment or for your departmental assessment. I have left spaces between the questions to write down your answers, or you can have your thoughts on separate sheet of paper. There is obviously no right or wrong answer to these questions, they are for you to assess where you are and what else you need to do to improve your effectiveness.

Questions for Director/Manager of Food Service

1. How long have you been at your current facility, or is this a new environment for you, and how well are you doing with all the roles and responsibilities of the position?

2. If you have been at your current facility for over a year, how well did you do at your last certification or complaint survey? If there are areas that you had deficiencies that need improvement, are you following your plan of correction to attain the goals you set for the needed improvement(s)?

3. Do you know that F812 is amongst the top ten (10) deficiencies in nursing homes/ skilled nursing facilities deficiencies? F812 is titled "Food Procurement, Store/ Prepare/Serve – Sanitary" in the Food and Nutrition Services Regulatory Groupings? How much monitoring do you engage your staff to do to establish compliance with your parts of the regulations?.

4. Do you have regular department meetings with your staff to assess and address staff issues and concerns, maintain team work, and also to use that opportunity to go over some of your most important policies and procedures?

5. How well do you keep abreast of the regulations for Food and Nutrition Services?

6. Are you and your staff ready for your upcoming survey, and do you take steps for your department to stay survey ready 365 days a year?

F-Tags For Food Service Director/Manager
F800
(Rev. 173, Issued: 11-22-17, Effective: 11-28-17, Implementation: 11-28-17)
§483.60 Food and nutrition services.

The facility must provide each resident with a nourishing, palatable, well-balanced diet that meets his or her daily nutritional and special dietary needs, taking into consideration the preferences of each resident.

INTENT §483.60 – To ensure that facility staff support the nutritional well-being of the residents while respecting an individual's right to make choices about his or her diet.

GUIDANCE §483.60

This requirement expects that there is ongoing communication and coordination among and between staff within all departments to ensure that the resident assessment, care plan and actual food and nutrition services meet each resident's daily nutritional and dietary needs and choices.

While it may be challenging to meet every resident's individual preferences, incorporating a resident's preferences and dietary needs will ensure residents are offered meaningful choices in meals/diets that are nutritionally adequate and satisfying to the individual. Reasonable efforts to accommodate these choices and preferences must be addressed by facility staff.

F801
(Rev. 207; Issued: 09-30-22; Effective: 09-30-22; Implementation: 10-01-22)
§483.60(a) Staffing

The facility must employ sufficient staff with the appropriate competencies and skills sets to carry out the functions of the food and nutrition service, taking into consideration resident assessments, individual plans of care and the number, acuity and diagnoses of the facility's resident population in accordance with the facility assessment required at §483.70(e)

This includes:

§483.60(a)(1) A qualified dietitian or other clinically qualified nutrition professional either full-time, part-time, or on a consultant basis. A qualified dietitian or other clinically qualified nutrition professional is one who—

> (i) **Holds a bachelor's or higher degree granted by a regionally accredited college or university in the United States (or an equivalent foreign**

degree) with completion of the academic requirements of a program in nutrition or dietetics accredited by an appropriate national accreditation organization recognized for this purpose.

(ii)   Has completed at least 900 hours of supervised dietetics practice under the supervision of a registered dietitian or nutrition professional.

(iii)   Is licensed or certified as a dietitian or nutrition professional by the State in which the services are performed. In a State that does not provide for licensure or certification, the individual will be deemed to have met this requirement if he or she is recognized as a "registered dietitian" by the Commission on Dietetic Registration or its successor organization, or meets the requirements of paragraphs (a)(1)(i) and (ii) of this section.

(iv)   For dietitians hired or contracted with prior to November 28, 2016, meets these requirements no later than 5 years after November 28, 2016 or as required by state law.

§483.60(a)(2) If a qualified dietitian or other clinically qualified nutrition professional is not employed full-time, the facility must designate a person to serve as the director of food and nutrition services.

(i)   The director of food and nutrition services must at a minimum meet one of the following qualifications—

A. A certified dietary manager; or
B. A certified food service manager; or
C. Has similar national certification for food service management and safety from a national certifying body; or
D. Has an associate's or higher degree in food service management or in hospitality, if the course study includes food service or restaurant management, from an accredited institution of higher learning; or
E. Has 2 or more years of experience in the position of director of food and nutrition services in a nursing facility setting and has completed a course of study in food safety and management, by no later than October 1, 2023, that includes topics integral to managing dietary operations including, but not limited to, foodborne illness, sanitation procedures, and food purchasing/receiving; and

(ii)   In States that have established standards for food service managers or dietary managers, meets State requirements for food service managers or dietary managers, and

(iii) **Receives frequently scheduled consultations from a qualified dietitian or other clinically qualified nutrition professional.**

INTENT §483.60 (a)(1)-(2) – To ensure there is sufficient and qualified staff with the appropriate competencies and skill sets to carry out food and nutrition services.

DEFINITIONS §483.60(a)(1)-(2)

"Full-time" means working 35 or more hours a week.

"Part-time" employees typically work fewer hours in a day or during a work week than full-time employees. The U.S. Department of Labor, Bureau of Statistics uses a definition of 34 or fewer hours a week as part-time work. Part-time workers may also be those who only work during certain parts of the year.

"Consultants" means an individual who gives professional advice or services. They are generally not direct employees of the facility and may work either full or part-time.

GUIDANCE §483.60(a)(1)-(2)

In addition, cite F801 if staff, specifically the qualified dietitian or other clinically nutrition professional did not carry out the functions of the food and nutrition services. While these functions may be defined by facility management, at a minimum they should include, but are not limited to:

- Assessing the nutritional needs of residents;
- Developing and evaluating regular and therapeutic diets, including texture of foods and liquids, to meet the specialized needs of residents;
- Developing and implementing person centered education programs involving food and nutrition services for all facility staff;
- Overseeing the budget and purchasing of food and supplies, and food preparation, service and storage; and
- Participating in the quality assurance and performance improvement (QAPI), as described in §483.75, when food and nutrition services are involved.

The qualified dietitian or other clinically qualified nutrition professional can decide to oversee and delegate some of the activities listed above to the director of food and nutrition services.

Remarks

Remark – dietitians, you can see how important your role is to the facility as a whole. The third bullet above is very informative about your role in educating facility staffs about person-centered care for residents. You will need to coordinate with the staff development and with the administrator and director of nursing for effective implementation of this educational in-services program. To reinforce the point that resident mealtime experience contributes to the residents' quality of life. Enhancing the mealtime experience to that of a quality and pleasant experience adds to the improvement of the residents' quality of life.

F802
(Rev. 173, Issued: 11-22-17, Effective: 11-28-17, Implementation: 11-28-17)
§483.60(a) Staffing

The facility must employ sufficient staff with the appropriate competencies and skills sets to carry out the functions of the food and nutrition service, taking into consideration resident assessments, individual plans of care and the number, acuity and diagnoses of the facility's resident population in accordance with the facility assessment required at §483.70(e).

§483.60(a)(3) Support staff.

The facility must provide sufficient support personnel to safely and effectively carry out the functions of the food and nutrition service.

§483.60(b) A member of the Food and Nutrition Services staff must participate on the interdisciplinary team as required in § 483.21(b)(2)(ii).

DEFINITION §483.60(a)(3)-(b)

"Sufficient support personnel" means having enough dietary and food and nutrition staff to safely carry out all of the functions of the food and nutrition services. This does not include staff, such as licensed nurses, nurse aides or paid feeding assistants, involved in assisting residents with eating.

F803
(Rev. 173, Issued: 11-22-17, Effective: 11-28-17, Implementation: 11-28-17)
§483.60(c) Menus and nutritional adequacy.

Menus must—

§483.60(c)(1) Meet the nutritional needs of residents in accordance with established national guidelines;

§483.60(c)(2) Be prepared in advance;

§483.60(c)(3) Be followed;

§483.60(c)(4) Reflect, based on a facility's reasonable efforts, the religious, cultural and ethnic needs of the resident population, as well as input received from residents and resident groups;

§483.60(c)(5) Be updated periodically;

§483.60(c)(6) Be reviewed by the facility's dietitian or other clinically qualified nutrition professional for nutritional adequacy; and

§483.60(c)(7) Nothing in this paragraph should be constructed to limit the resident's right to make personal dietary choices.

INTENT §483.60(c)(1)-(7) – To assure that menus are developed and prepared to meet resident choices including their nutritional, religious, cultural, and ethnic needs while using established national guidelines.

DEFINITIONS §483.60(c)(1)-(7)

"**Reasonable effort**" means assessing individual resident needs and preferences and demonstrating actions to meet those needs and preferences, including reviewing availability of procurement sources of such food items, identifying preparation methods and approaches, and determining whether purchasing and serving such items can occur.

"**Periodically**" means that a facility should update its menus to accommodate their changing resident population or resident needs as determined by their facility assessment. See F838. This includes ethnic, cultural, or religious factors that may potentially affect the care provided by the facility, including, but not limited to, activities and food and nutrition services.

GUIDANCE §483.60(c)(1-7)

The facility must make reasonable efforts to provide food that is appetizing to and culturally appropriate for residents. This means learning the residents' needs and preferences and responding to them. For residents with dementia or other barriers or challenges to expressing their preferences, facility staff should document the steps taken to learn what those preferences are.

It is not required that there be individualized menus for all residents; however, alternatives aligned with individual needs and preference should be available if the primary menu or immediate selections for a particular meal are not to a resident's liking.

F804
(Rev. 173, Issued: 11-22-17, Effective: 11-28-17, Implementation: 11-28-17)
§483.60(d) Food and drink
Each resident receives and the facility provides—
§483.60(d)(1) Food prepared by methods that conserve nutritive value, flavor, and appearance;
§483.60(d)(2) Food and drink that is palatable, attractive, and at a safe and appetizing temperature.

INTENT §483.60(d)(1)-(2) – To assure that the nutritive value of food is not compromised and destroyed because of prolonged:

1. Food storage, light, and air exposure; or
2. Cooking of foods in a large volume of water; or
3. Holding on steam table.

DEFINITIONS §483.60(d)(1)-(2)

"Food attractiveness" refers to the appearance of the food when **served** to residents.

"Food palatability" refers to the taste and/or flavor of the food.

"Proper (safe and appetizing) temperature" means both appetizing to the resident and minimizing the risk for scalding and burns.

Remarks

Remarks – CMS is stressing the fact that the food served to the resident must be palatable, attractive, and an appetizing temperature based on the type of food as the satisfaction pf the residents must be one of the major considerations. Food temperature must meet standards to avoid the risk of scalding and burns.

F805
(Rev. 173, Issued: 11-22-17, Effective: 11-28-17, Implementation: 11-28-17)
§483.60(d) Food and drink
Each resident receives and the facility provides—
§483.60(d)(3) Food prepared in a form designed to meet individual needs.

F806
(Rev. 173, Issued: 11-22-17, Effective: 11-28-17, Implementation: 11-28-17)
§483.60(d) Food and Drink
Each resident receives and the facility provides—
§483.60(d)(4) Food that accommodates resident allergies, intolerances, and preferences;

§483.60(d)(5) Appealing options of similar nutritive value to residents who choose not to eat food that is initially served or who request a different meal choice; and

GUIDANCE §483.60 (d)(4)-(5)

Facilities should be aware of each resident's allergies, intolerances, and preferences, and provide an appropriate alternative. A food substitute should be consistent with the usual and/or ordinary food items provided by the facility. For example, the facility may, instead of grapefruit juice, substitute another citrus juice or vitamin C rich juice the resident likes.

F807
(Rev. 173, Issued: 11-22-17, Effective: 11-28-17, Implementation: 11-28-17)
§483.60(d) Food and drink
Each resident receives and the facility provides—

§483.60(d)(6) Drinks, including water and other liquids consistent with resident needs and preferences and sufficient to maintain resident hydration.

Remarks

Remarks – the GUIDANCE addresses the need for hydration. It is informative here that staff should be aware that proper hydration alone is critical to nutrition among nursing home residents. For individuals that may not receive adequate fluids it is possible to put some of those residents at risk of negative outcomes such as urinary tract infections, pneumonia, decubitus ulcers, skin infections, confusion and disorientation may be associated to lack of fluids.

F808
(Rev. 173, Issued: 11-22-17, Effective: 11-28-17, Implementation: 11-28-17)
§483.60(e)Therapeutic Diets
§483.60(e)(1) Therapeutic diets must be prescribed by the attending physician.
§483.60(e)(2) The attending physician may delegate to a registered or licensed dietitian the task of prescribing a resident's diet, including a therapeutic diet, to the extent allowed by State law.

INTENT §483.60(e)(1)-(2) – To assure that resident receive and consume foods in the appropriate form and/or the appropriate nutritive content as prescribed by a physician, and/or assessed by the interdisciplinary team to support the resident's treatment, plan of care, in accordance with his her goals and preferences.

GUIDANCE §483.60(e)(1)-(2)

If the residents' attending physician delegates this task he or she must supervise the dietitian and remains responsible for the resident's care even if the task is delegated. The physician would be able to modify a diet order with a subsequent order, if necessary.

NOTE: The term "attending physician" or "physician" also includes a non-physician provider (physician assistant, nurse practitioner, or clinical nurse specialist) involved in the management of the resident's care.

DEFINITIONS §483.60(e)(1)-(2)

"**Therapeutic Diet**" means a diet ordered by a physician or delegated registered or licensed dietitian as part of treatment for a disease or clinical condition, or to eliminate or decrease specific nutrients in the diet, (e.g. sodium) or to increase specific nutrients in the diet (e.g., potassium), or to provide food the resident is able to eat (e.g., a mechanically altered diet).

"**Mechanically altered diet**" means one in which the texture of a diet is altered. When the texture is modified, the type of texture modification must be specified and part of the physicians' or delegated registered or licensed dietitian order.

F809
(Rev. 173, Issued: 11-22-17, Effective: 11-28-17, Implementation: 11-28-17)
§483.60(f) Frequency of Meals
§483.60(f)(1) Each resident must receive and the facility must provide at least three meals daily, at regular times comparable to normal mealtimes in the community or in accordance with resident needs, preferences, requests, and plan of care.

§483.60(f)(2) There must be no more than 14 hours between a substantial evening meal and breakfast the following day, except when a nourishing snack is served at bedtime, up to 16 hours may elapse between a substantial evening meal and breakfast the following day if a resident group agrees to this meal span.

§483.60(f)(3) Suitable, nourishing alternative meals and snacks must be provided to residents who want to eat at nom-traditional times or outside of scheduled meal service times, consistent with the resident plan of care.

DEFINITIONS §483.60(f)(1)-(3)

A "**Nourishing snack**" means items from the basic food groups, either singly or in combination with each other.

"**Suitable and nourishing alternative meals and snacks**" means that when an alternate meal or snack is provided, it is of similar nutritive value as the meal or snack offered at the normally scheduled time and consistent with the resident plan of care.

Remarks

Remarks – based on the GUIDANCE to surveyors, CMS stated that facilities should recognize resident's needs, preferences and requests for alternate or substitute meals, and alternate times that some residents may want to eat their meals. Facilities should make accommodation for those alternate times. CMS also acknowledge that as much as facilities must accommodate these preferences and alternate meal times for some residents if requested, it does not mean that facilities are required to have a 24-hour-a-day full service food operation or on-site chef. Suitable alternatives can be made.

It is also important that the facility have a system providing possible alternative to the main menu item so the residents can make a selection ahead to receive the alternative food item when the tray is delivered. When residents request alternate food items after the food tray has been delivered to the unit and other residents are eating their meal in the dining room, and residents have to wait for the alternate item to be delivered that does not give a pleasant mealtime experience for that resident or those residents.

F810
(Rev. 173, Issued: 11-22-17, Effective: 11-28-17, Implementation: 11-28-17)
§483.60(g) Assistive devices

The facility must provide special eating equipment and utensils for residents who need them and appropriate assistance to ensure that the resident can use the assistive devices when consuming meals and snacks.

GUIDANCE §483.60(g)

The facility must provide appropriate assistive devices to residents who need them to maintain or improve their ability to eat or drink independently, for example, improving poor grasp by enlarging silverware handles with foam padding, aiding residents with impaired coordination or tremor by installing plate guards, or specialized cups. The facility must also provide the appropriate staff assistance to ensure that these residents can use the assistive devices when eating or drinking.

Remarks

Remark - If you are wondering why I skipped F811, here, I did so because the Director of Nursing has the responsibility for Feeding Assistants, if and when a facility uses feeding assistants to help feed or assist residents with their meals.

F812
(Rev. 211; Issued: 02-03-23; Effective: 10-21-22; Implementation: 10-24-22)
§483.60(i) Food safety requirements.

The facility must—

§483.60(i)(1) – Procure food from sources approved or considered satisfactory by federal, state or local authorities.

(i)   **This may include food items obtained directly from local producers, subject to applicable State and local laws or regulations.**

(ii)   **This provision does not prohibit or prevent facilities from using produce grown in facility gardens, subject to compliance with applicable safe growing and food-handling practices.**

(iii)   **This provision does not preclude residents from consuming foods not procured by the facility.**

§483.60(i)(2) – Store, prepare, distribute and serve food in accordance with professional standards for food service safety.

INTENT §483.60(i)(1)-(2) – "To ensure that the facility:

- Obtains food for resident consumption from sources approved or considered satisfactory by Federal, State or local authorities;
- Follows proper sanitation and food handling practices to prevent the outbreak of foodborne illness. Safe food handling for the prevention of foodborne illnesses begins when food is received from the vendor and continues throughout the facility's food handling processes; and
- Ensures food safety is maintained when implementing various culture change initiatives such as when serving buffet style from a portable steam table, or during a potluck.

DEFINITIONS §483.60(i)-(2)

The following definitions are provided to clarify terms related to professional standards for food service safety, sanitary conditions and the prevention of foodborne illness. Foodborne illness refers to illness caused by the ingestion of contaminated food or beverages.

"Critical Control Point" means a specific point, procedure, or step in food preparation and serving process at which control can be exercised to reduce, eliminate, or prevent the possibility of a food safety hazard.

"Cross-contamination" means the transfer of harmful substances or disease—causing microorganisms to food by hands, food contact surfaces, sponges, cloth towels, or utensils which are not cleaned after touching raw food, and then touched ready-to-eat foods. Cross-contamination can also occur when raw food touches or drips onto cooked or ready-to-eat foods.

"Danger Zone" means temperatures above 41 degrees Fahrenheit (F) and below 135 degrees F that allow the rapid growth of pathogenic microorganisms that can cause foodborne illness. Potentially Hazardous Foods (PHF) or Time/Temperature Control for Safety (TCS) Foods held in the danger zone for more than 4 hours (if being prepared from ingredients at ambient temperature) or 6 hours (if cooked and cooled) may cause a foodborne illness outbreak if consumed.

"Dry Storage" means storing/maintaining dry foods (canned goods, flour, sugar, etc.) and supplies (disposable dishware, napkins, and kitchen cleaning supplies).

"Food Contamination" means the unintended presence of potentially harmful substances, including, but not limited to microorganisms, chemicals, or physical objects in food.

"Food Preparation" means the series of operational processes involved in preparing foods for serving, such as: washing, thawing, mixing ingredients, cutting, slicing, diluting concentrates, cooking, pureeing, blending, cooling, and reheating.

"Food Distribution" means the processes involved in getting food to the resident. This may include holding foods hot on the steam table or under refrigeration for cold temperature control, dispensing food portions for individual residents, family style and dining room service, or delivering meals to residents' rooms or dining areas, etc. When meals are assembled in the kitchen and then delivered to residents' rooms or dining areas to be distributed, covering foods is appropriate, either individually or in a mobile food caret.

"Food Service" means the processes involved in actively serving food to the resident. When actively serving residents in a dining room or outside a resident's room where trained staff are serving food/beverage choices directly from a mobile food cart or steam table, there is no need for food to be covered. However, food should be covered when traveling a distance (i.e. down a hallway, to a different unit or floor).

"Potentially Hazardous Food (PHF)" or **"Time/Temperature Control for Safety (TCS) Food"** means food that requires time/temperature control for safety to limit the growth of pathogens (i.e., bacterial or viral organisms capable of causing a disease or toxin formation).

"**Storage**" refers to the retention of food (before and after preparation) and associated dry goods.

GUIDANCE §483.60(i)(1)-(2) (This is abridged form of the guidance; refer to State Operations Manual Appendix PP for full and detailed content of the guidance.) This guidance content has very detailed information about food contamination, about food borne illnesses, food distribution, food storage, employee health hair restraints/ coverings, food service, food distribution, etc. see also remarks below)

Nursing home residents risk serious complications from foodborne illness as a result of their compromised health status. Unsafe food handling practices represent a potential source of pathogen exposure for residents. Sanitary conditions must be present in health care food service settings to promote safe food handling. CMS recognizes the US Food and Drug Administration's (FDA) Food Code and the Centers for Disease Control and Prevention's (CDC) food safety guidance as national standards to procure, store, prepare, distribute, and serve food in long term care facilities in a safe and sanitary manner.

Effective food safety systems involve identifying hazards at specific points during food handling and preparation, and identifying how the hazards can be prevented, reduced or eliminated. It is important to focus attention on the risks that are associated with foodborne illness by identifying critical control points (CCPs) in the food preparation processes that, if not controlled, might result in food safety hazards. Some operational steps that are critical to control in facilities to prevent or eliminate food safety hazards are thawing, cooking, cooling, holding, reheating of foods, and employee hygienic practices:

- Web sites for additional information regarding safe food handling to minimize the potential for foodborne illness include" National Food Safety Information Network's Gateway to Government Food Safety Information at http://www. FoodSafety.gov;
- United States Food & Drug Administration Food Code Web site at https://www. fda.gov/food/fda-food-code/food-code-2017"

Remarks

Remark - To give you an idea of the details covered in this F812 tag section, I am listing below the topics that you will find in the State Operations Manual (SOM) Appendix PP GUIDANCE for this F-tag, as CMS delineates detailed description of what you need to know about each topic area. These topic headings listed below are essential for you to effectively and successfully operate your Food Service Department. Below is the list of topics and detailed content in the F812 Tag; refer to the State Operations Manual Appendix PP for F-tag 812 for the detailed information on the topics listed below. in the section in the SOM.

- Food contamination – there are three (3) categories identified: Biological Contamination; Chemical Contamination; and Physical Contamination
- Potential Factors Implicated in Foodborne Illnesses – these include Poor Personal Hygiene, Inadequate Cooking and Improper Holding Temperatures, Contaminated Equipment, Unsafe Food Sources
- Employee Health
- Hand Washing, Gloves, and Antimicrobial Gel,
- Hair Restraints/Jewelry/Nail Polish
- Food Receiving and Storage
- Personal Refrigerators
- Dry Food Storage
- Refrigerated Storage
- Safe Food Preparation
  - Cross-Contamination
  - Thawing
  - Final Cooking Temperatures
  - Reheating Foods
  - Cooling
  - Modified Consistency
  - Eggs
- Food Distribution
- Food Service
- Food preparation or service area problems/risks to avoid
- Snacks
- Special Events
- Potluck Events
- Nursing Home Gardens
- Transported Foods
- Ice
- Refrigeration

- Personal Refrigerators
- Equipment and Utensil Cleaning and Sanitation
- Machine Washing and Sanitizing
- Manual Washing and Sanitizing
- Cleaning Fixed Equipment

F813
(Rev. 173, Issued: 11-22-17, Effective: 11-28-17, Implementation: 11-28-17)
§483.60(i) Food Safety Requirements
The facility must
§483.60(i)(3) Have a policy regarding use and storage of foods brought to residents by family and other visitors to ensure safe and sanitary storage, handling, and consumption.

GUIDANCE §483.60(i)(3)

The facility must have a policy regarding food brought to residents by family and other visitors. The policy must also include ensuring facility staff assists the resident in accessing and consuming the food, if the resident is not able to do so on his or her own. The facility also is responsible for storing food brought in by family or visitors in a way that is either separate or easily distinguished from facility food.

The facility has the responsibility to help family and visitors understand safe food handling practices (such as safe cooling/reheating processes, hot/cold holding temperatures, preventing cross contamination, hand hygiene, etc.). If the facility is assisting family or visitors with reheating or other preparation activities, facility staff must use safe food handling practices.

F814
(Rev. 173, Issued: 11-22-17, Effective: 11-28-17, Implementation: 11-28-17)
§483.60(i) Food Safety Requirements
The facility must—
§483.60(i)(4)- Dispose of garbage and refuse properly.

Next sets of F-Tag here are Quality of Life – F675; Quality of Care – F684; and Nutrition/Hydration Status Maintenance – Quality of Care.

Remarks

Remarks - To reinforce the importance of the inter-relatedness of the disciplines and the departments, I want to buttress that point here by including **F675** – "Quality of Life", and **F684 and F692** "Quality of Care" in the section of the Food Service Director/ Manager. I am providing here a brief and abridged form of the important fundamentals of "Quality of Life" and "Quality of Care" F-Tags. As Food Service Director/Manager you need to know your role in the quality of life and quality of care of the residents. If you need additional information about the Quality of Life and/or Quality of Care, you can refer to those F-tags in other areas of the workbook.

F675
(Rev. 211; Issued: 102-03-23; Effective: 10-21-22; Implementation:10-24-22)
§483.24 Quality of life

Quality of life is a fundamental principle that applies to all care and services provided to facility residents. Each resident must receive and the facility must provide the necessary care and services to attain or maintain the highest practicable physical, mental, and psychosocial well-being, consistent with the resident's comprehensive assessment and plan of care.

INTENT

The intent of this requirement is to specify the facility's responsibility to create and sustain an environment that humanizes and individuals each resident's quality of life by:

- Ensuring all staff, across all shifts and departments, understand the principles of quality of life, and honor and support these principles for each resident; and
- Ensuring that the care and services provided are person-centered, and honor and support each resident's preferences, choices, values and beliefs.

DEFINITIONS §483.24

"Person Centered Care" – For this purposes of this subpart, person-centered care means to focus on the resident as the locus of control and support the resident in making their own choices and having control over their daily lives,

"**Pervasive**" For the purposes of this guidance, pervasive means spread through or embedded within every part of something.

"**Quality of Life**" refers to an individual's sense of well-being, level of satisfaction with life and feeling of self-worth and self-esteem. For nursing home residents, this includes a basic sense of satisfaction with oneself, the environment, the care received, the accomplishments of desired goals, and control over one's life." Adopted from the 1986 Institute of Medicine (IOM) published report "Improving the Quality of Care in Nursing Homes." Located at: https://www.ncbi.nih.gov/books/NBK217548/#ddd00037

F684
(Rev. 173, Issued: 11-22-17, Effective: 11-28-17, Implementation: 11-28-17)
§483.25 Quality of care

Quality of care is a fundamental principle that applies to all treatment and care provided to facility residents. Based on the comprehensive assessment of a resident, the facility must ensure that residents receive treatment and care in accordance with professional standards of practice, the comprehensive person-centered care plan, and the residents' choices, including but not limited to the following:

INTENT

To ensure facilities identify and provide needed care and services that are resident centered, in accordance with the resident's preferences, goals for care and professional standards of practice that will meet each resident's physical, mental, and psychosocial needs.

DEFINITIONS

"**Highest practicable physical, mental, and psychosocial well-being**" is defined as the highest possible level of functioning and well-being, limited by the individual's recognized pathology and normal aging process. Highest practicable is determined through the comprehensive resident assessment and by recognizing and competently and thoroughly addressing the physical, mental or psychosocial needs of the individual.

"**Hospice Care**" means a comprehensive set of services described in Section 1861(dd)(1) of the Act, identified and coordinated by an interdisciplinary group (IDG) to provide for the physical, psychosocial, spiritual, and emotional needs of a terminally ill patient and/or family members, as delineated in a specific patient plan of care. (42 CFR §418.3)

"**Palliative care**" means patient and family-centered care that optimizes quality of life by anticipating, preventing, and treating suffering. Palliative care throughout the continuum of illness involves addressing physical, intellectual, emotional, social, and spiritual needs and to facilitate patient autonomy, access to information, and choice. (§418.3)

"**Terminally ill**" means that the individual has a medical prognosis that his or her life expectancy is 6 months or less if the illness runs its normal course. (§418.3)

F692
(Rev. 173, Issued: 11-22-17, Effective: 11-28-17, Implementation: 11-28-17)
§483.25(g) Assisted nutrition and hydration.

(Includes naso-gastric and gastrostomy tubes, both percutaneous endoscopic gastrostomy and percutaneous endoscopic jejunostomy, and enteral fluids). Based on a resident's comprehensive assessment, the facility must ensure that a resident—

§483.25(g)(1) Maintain acceptable parameters of nutritional status, such as usual body weight or desirable body weight range and electrolyte balance, unless the resident's clinical condition demonstrates that this is not possible or resident preferences indicate otherwise;

§483.25(g)(2) Is offered sufficient fluid intake to maintain proper hydration and health;

§483.25(g)(3) Is offered a therapeutic diet when there is a nutritional problem and the health care provider orders a therapeutic diet.

INTENT §483.25(g)

The intent of this requirement is that the resident maintains, to the extent possible, acceptable parameters of nutritional and hydration status and that the facility:

- Provides nutritional and hydration care and services to each resident, consistent with the resident's comprehensive assessment;

- Recognizes, evaluates, and addresses the needs of every resident, including but not limited to, the resident at risk or already experiencing impaired nutrition and hydration; and
- Provides a therapeutic diet that takes into account the resident's clinical condition, and preferences, when there is a nutritional indication.

DEFINITIONS

Definitions are provided to clarify clinical terms related to nutritional status.

"Acceptable parameters of nutritional status" refers to factors that reflect that an individual's nutritional status is adequate, relative to his/her overall condition and prognosis, such as weight, food/fluid intake, and pertinent laboratory values.

"Artificial nutrition and hydration" are medical treatments and refer to nutrition that is provided through routes other than the usual oral route, tyupically by placing a tube directly into the stomach, the intestine or a vein.

"Clinically significant" refers to effects, results, or consequences that materially affect or are likely to affect an individual's physical, mental, or psychosocial well-being either positively by preventing, stabilizing, or improving a condition or reducing a risk \, or negatively by exacerbating, causing, or contributing to a symptom, illness, or decline in status.

"Dietary supplement" refers to herbal and alternative products that are not regulated by the Food and Drug Administration and their composition is not standardized. Dietary supplements must be labeled as such and must not be represented for use as a conventional food or as the sole item of a meal or the diet.

"Health Care Provider" includes a physician, physician assistant, nurse practitioner, or clinical nurse specialist, or a qualified dietitian or other qualified nutrition professional acting within their state scope of practice and to whom the attending physician has delegated the task. For issues related to delegation to dietitians, refer to §483.60(e)(2), F808

"Nutritional status" includes both nutrition and hydration status.

"Nutritional Supplements" refers to products that are used to complement a resident's dietary needs (e.g. calorie or nutrient dense drinks, total parenteral products, enteral products, and meal replacement products).

"Therapeutic diet" refers to a diet ordered by a physician or other delegated provider that is part of the treatment for a disease or clinical condition, to eliminate, decrease, or increase certain substances in the diet (e.g. sodium or potassium), or to provide mechanically altered food when indicated.

"Tube feeding" refers to the delivery of nutrients through a feeding tube directly into the stomach, duodenum, or jejunum. It is also referred to as enteral feeding.

Chapter 11

PRACTICAL TIPS FOR DIRECTOR/MANAGER OF FOOD SERVICE AND CASE STUDY

Tips

- The Food Service Department staff – directors, managers, supervisors, food service aides and others must know the regulations that relate to your areas of responsibility. This will enable you to provide the needed services for the residents, maintain regulatory compliance, and ensure the quality of care and services. It will also make you survey ready for whenever surveyors walk through your doors.

- So you are aware, whenever surveyors come to your facility to conduct surveys, one or two surveyors immediately proceed to the kitchen to briefly observe your operation, the cleanliness of the kitchen, infection control protocols, your freezer and refrigerator temperature logs, other logs, etc. and other areas of interest to them, in the kitchen.

- Conduct Environment of Care (EOC) Rounds at minimum weekly. The Food Service Director and Supervisors must be part of the EOC Rounds team.

- Temperature logs for the freezer and for the walk-in refrigerators must be retained for proof that the temperatures for the equipment are maintained at the required levels.

- Logs also for the dish machine must also be retained so facility can prove that the wash and rinse cycle were and are operating properly as required.

- Food distribution to residents must be maintained at the proper temperature levels, both cold food and hot food.

- Food in the walk-in refrigerators must be labeled and dated, because there should be no food beyond the stale date.

- The cycle menus must be available for review.

- The kitchen must be kept clean at all times.

- All staff must always wear or have appropriate head coverings.

- Infection control protocols for the kitchen must be maintained at all times.

- Stay abreast of regulations for Food and Nutrition Services, Quality of Care and Services, and Quality of Life.

- Have monthly general staff meetings to establish and maintain the environment for departmental communication and teamwork.

- Have regular meetings also with department supervisors to help mentor them and develop their supervisory skills when needed for growth and department cohesiveness. Also provide one-to-one mentoring as you see fit.

- Surveyors also observe storage of dry goods in the kitchen, so store dry goods appropriately.

CASE STUDY

DISCLAIMER: This case study is fictional – fictional names of skilled nursing facilities and/or nursing homes, fictional situations and fictional stories. The names, characters and incidents portrayed in the case studies are fictional, and no identification with persons (living or dead) and with places or with products should be assumed or inferred.

CASE STUDY

One early Tuesday morning, five (5) State Surveyors showed up at XYZ Skilled Nursing Facility to conduct the annual certification survey. The surveyors arrived at the facility at 7:15 AM. The Administrator and the Food Service Director were on their way to the office at this time, so they were not available when the surveyors arrived. The Director of Nursing (DON) welcomed the surveyors, and had them situated at the facility conference room. The Administrative Assistant and DON called the administrator to let him know that surveyors were at the facility. The survey Team Leader informed the DON that they were at the facility for the facility's annual certification survey. The Team Leader dispatched one (1) surveyor to the kitchen for immediate observation of the kitchen operation. The other four (4) surveyors planned to go to the units to observe breakfast meal time on the units as their first assignment.

The surveyor, whose assignment was to go to the kitchen, was escorted to the kitchen by a nurse manager. As the food service director was on her way to the office, the surveyor met with the food service supervisor to explain that she was there for the annual certification survey. When the surveyor went to the kitchen, she observed the staff at "tray line" assembling and getting breakfast on the tray line to be taken to the units. The surveyor noticed something unusual at the tray line conveyor belt, and the surveyor asked the food service supervisor, "Why are you serving food on paper plates?" The food service supervisor answered: "the dish machine was down yesterday, and we have called the repair people, so we did not want to take the chance to use the china plates, because we don't know when they will finish repairing the machine." The surveyor's next question was "So did you send communication to the units to let the unit managers and the residents know that the residents will receive their breakfast meal on paper plates and plastic cutlery instead of the china plates?" The food service supervisor responded, "Oh no, I forgot. I am going to call the nurse managers right away, so they can let the residents know, and extend our apologies. And we will keep them informed as the repairs progress. I hope they can fix the dish machine soon so the residents can eat their lunch on the usual china plates as they are accustomed to." The surveyor then requested to see the dish machine log for the past month. The log reflected some inconsistencies in the temperatures for the wash cycle and also for the rinse cycle.

The surveyor then proceeded to the walk-in refrigerators to check the temperature logs and the foods inside the walk-in refrigerators to see if foods were labelled with names of food and dates. The surveyor asked to see the temperature logs for the previous months.

The Food Service Director arrived at the office soon thereafter, and took over from the food service supervisor. So the surveyor continued discussions with her, the food service director, asking questions about her concerns. The surveyor continued her brief "walk-through" of the kitchen operations, but she had to let the survey Team Leader know her immediate findings about the kitchen thus far.

EXERCISES TO DO

A. List the concerns you identify which you believe the surveyor has shared with the Food Service Director thus far.

B. For your No. 1 concern, list below what your assessment of the failure or non-compliance was and how you will correct the system and address the problem so it does not happen again.

C. What is your concern # 2? What system needs to be put in place as corrective measure?

D. What is your concern # 3 if any? What system needs to be put in place as corrective measure if any?

E. Can you identify which F-tags or general Topic areas contributed to this non-compliance or failure to follow facility policy based on the regulation?

F. One of the problems/issues in long term care is survey readiness. Do you have a plan for survey readiness?

PART

6

Chapter 12

NURSE MANAGERS & CERTIFIED NURSING ASSISTANTS/CERTIFIED NURSE AIDES – ROLES AND F-TAG FOCUS THROUGH THE DIRECTOR OF NURSING

Questions for Nurse Managers and F-Tags Focus

As direct-caregivers - nurse managers, nursing supervisors, and certified nurse aides/certified nursing assistants spend more time with the residents; providing the direct care and services the residents require. Consequently they influence the quality of care and services the residents receive, as well as the influence they have on the residents' mealtime experience. The DON obviously has ultimate responsibility for the nursing personnel, but due to the direct care and daily influence nurse managers, nursing supervisors, and nurse aides/nursing assistants have on the residents daily lives, I made a decision to have a separate chapter for their roles and F-tags. I consider these direct caregivers members of the same team, who provide the quality of care, quality of life and safety of the residents.

I am listing a few questions for the Nurse Managers. These are self-assessment questions for reflection and to determine where you are and where you may want to be in the areas of your roles and responsibilities. You can use the space between the questions to provide the answers to the questions or you can use a separate sheet of paper.

Questions for Nurse Managers:

1. How will you rate your clinical skill sets (from 1 – 10, with 1 being the least) for the long term care environment and why did you give yourself that rating? If you need help in this area, in the performance of your duties, how do you go about seeking the help you want and need?

2. As supervisors, how will you rate your supervisory skill sets (from 1 – 10, with 1 being the least) within the long term care environment and with nurse aides, and why did you give yourself that rating? How is your working relationship between you and the certified nursing assistants/certified nurse aides?

3. Understanding the inter-relatedness of the departments, and the interdisciplinary nature of the operations in long term care, are your communication and management skills meeting the expectation and contribution towards the residents clinical needs?

4. Do you provide official or unofficial mentorship for the (your) certified nursing assistants/nurse aides at your facility to guide them as they perform their direct care duties if and when needed?

5. How well did your unit do in your last certification or complaint survey, and what are you currently doing to stay survey ready for your upcoming survey?

6. Do you participate in monitoring resident meal time, and how often do you monitor meal time?

7. Do you help the nurse aides with the residents' meal to ensure there is enough staff to help with residents meals?

8. How well are your assessment skills? Do you conduct assessment of your residents timely?

9. Care planning is super-important, how well do you make sure you develop and follow up with the 48-Hour care plan, quarterly annual, and other care plans that are needed for the residents care, such as resident change in condition?

F-tags for Nurse Managers/Supervisors for Certified Nursing Assistants/Nurse Aides

Nurse Managers, you will find that there are some more detailed F-Tags in this section, as you and the nursing assistants/nurse aides provide the connection between the residents and the kitchen staff particularly when there are issues and concerns with the residents' meal. You advocate for the residents when residents may need to substitute food items for their preferences or advocate for the residents to make things right during mealtime, and you help the facility help the residents have a pleasant mealtime experience. You have an awesome responsibility when it comes to residents' mealtime experience.

As nurse managers the facility leadership, both the administrator and director of nursing will expect you to be an important role model, teacher, and mentor to guide the process forward to make certain that your team provide the quality of care and services and contribute to a pleasant meal time experience for the residents. Your team(s) includes the nursing assistants/nurse aides, the direct caregivers who work on your units or floors.

F-Tags for Nurse Managers/Supervisors for Certified Nursing Assistants/Certified Nurse Aides
F550
(Rev. 173, Issued: 11-22-17, Effective: 11-28-17, Implementation: 11-28-17)
§483.10(a) Resident Rights.

The resident has a right to a dignified existence, self-determination, and communication with and access to persons and services inside and outside the facility, including those specified in this section.

§483.10(a)(1) A facility must treat each resident with respect and dignity and care for each resident in a manner and in an environment that promotes maintenance or enhancement of his or her quality of life, recognizing each resident's individuality. The facility must protect and promote the rights of the resident.

§483.10(a)(2) The facility must provide equal access to quality care regardless of diagnosis, severity of condition, or payment source. A facility must establish and maintain identical policies and practices regarding transfer, discharge, and the provision of services under the State plan for all residents regardless of payment source.

§483.10(b) Exercise of Rights.

The resident has the right to exercise his or her rights as a resident of the facility and as a citizen or resident of the United States.

§483.10(b)(1) The facility must ensure that the resident can exercise his or her rights without interference, coercion, discrimination, or reprisal from the facility.

§483.10(b)(2) The resident has the right to be free of interference, coercion, discrimination, and reprisal from the facility in exercising his or her rights and to be supported by the facility in the exercise of his or her rights as required under this subpart.

INTENT §483.10(a)-(b)(1)&(2)

All residents have the rights guaranteed to them under Federal and State laws and regulations. This regulation is intended to lay the foundation for the resident rights requirements in long-term care facilities. Each resident has the right to be treated with dignity and respect.. All activities and interactions with residents by any staff, temporary agency staff or volunteers must focus on assisting the resident in maintaining and enhancing his or her self-esteem and self-worth and incorporating the resident's, goals, preferences, and choices. When providing care and services, staff must respect each resident's individuality, as well as honor and value their input.

GUIDANCE §483.10(a)-(b)(1)&(2) (This is an abridged form of the guidance; refer to State Operations Manual Appendix PP for the full content of the guidance)

Examples of treating residents with dignity and respect include, but are not limited to:

- Encouraging and assisting residents to dress in their own clothes, rather than hospital-type gowns, and appropriate footwear for the time of day and individual preferences;
- Placing labels on each resident's clothing in a way that is inconspicuous and respects his or her dignity (for example, placing labeling on the inside of shoes and clothing or using a color coding system);
- Promoting resident independence and dignity while dining, such as avoiding:
  - Daily use of disposable cutlery and dishware;
  - Bibs or clothing protectors instead of napkins (except by resident choice);
  - Staff standing over residents while assisting them to eat;
  - Staff interacting/conversing only with each other rather than with residents while assisting with meals;
- Staff should address residents with the name or pronoun of the resident's choice, avoiding the use of labels for residents such as "feeders" or "walkers." Residents should not be excluded from conversations during activities or when care is being provided, nor should staff discuss residents in settings where others can overhear private or protected information or document in charts/electronic health records where others can see a resident's information;
- Refraining from practices demeaning to residents such as leaving urinary catheter bags uncovered, refusing to comply with a resident's request for bathroom assistance during meal times, and restricting residents from use of common areas open to the general public such as lobbies and restrooms, unless they are on transmission-based isolation precautions or are restricted according to their care planned needs."

F561
(Rev. 211; Issued: 02-03-23; Effective: 10-21-22; Implementation: 10-24-22)
§483.10(f) Self-determination.

The resident has the right to and the facility must promote and facilitate resident self-determination through support of resident choice, including but not limited to the rights specified in paragraphs (f)(1) through (11) of this section.

§483.10(f)(1) The resident has the right to choose activities, schedules (including sleeping and waking times), health care and providers of health care services consistent with his or her interests, assessments, and plan of care and other applicable provisions of this part.

§483.10(f)(2) The resident has a right to make choices about aspects of his or her life in the facility that are significant to the resident.

§483.10(f)(3) The resident has a right to interact with members of the community and participate in community activities both inside and outside the facility.

§483.10(f)(8) The resident has a right to participate in other activities, including social, religious, and community activities that do not interfere with the rights of other residents in the facility.

INTENT §483.10(f)(1)-(3) and (8)

The intent of this requirement is to ensure that each resident has the opportunity to exercise his or her autonomy regarding those things that are important in his or her life. This includes the residents' interests and preferences.

GUIDANCE §483.10(f)(1)-(3), (8) (This is an abridged form of the guidance; refer to the State Operations Manual Appendix PP for the full content of this guidance)

It is important for residents to have a choice about which activities they participate in, whether they are part of the formal activities program or self-directed. Additionally, a resident's needs and choices for how he or she spends time, both inside or outside the facility, should also be supported and accommodated, to the extent possible, including making transportation.

Residents have the right to choose their schedules, consistent with their interests, assessments, and care plans. This includes, but is not limited to, choices about the schedules that are important to the resident, such as waking, eating, bathing, and going to bed at night. Choices about schedules and ensuring that residents are able to get enough sleep, is an important contributor to overall health and well-being. Residents also have the right to choose health care schedules consistent with their interests and preferences, and information should be gathered to proactively assist residents with the fulfillment of their choices. Facilities must not develop a schedule for care, such as waking or bathing schedule, for staff convenience and without the input of the residents.

Remarks

Remark - For Nurse managers/supervisors, I am giving you **F-Tag - F584** because you and your teams are the direct caregivers to the residents, and you are constantly and consistently in the residents' presence and environment- in their rooms, in the dining rooms, in the lounge etc., so when the surroundings and atmosphere in the residents' rooms or in the dining rooms or other areas do not meet reasonable standard, it is your responsibility to ensure that the situation is reported to the appropriate department for corrective measures to be taken, and fix the problem.

F584
(Rev. 211; Issued: 02-03-23; Effective: 10-21-22; Implementation: 10-24-22)
§483.10(i) Safe Environment.

The resident has a right to a safe, clean, comfortable and homelike environment, including but not limited to receiving treatment and support for daily lining safely.

The facility must provide—

§483.10(i)(1) A safe, clean, comfortable, and homelike environment, allowing the resident to use his or her personal belongings to the extent possible.

> **(i)** **This includes ensuring that the resident can receive care and services safely and that the physical layout of the facility maximizes resident independence and does not pose a safety risk.**
>
> **(ii)** **The facility shall exercise reasonable care for the protection of the resident's property from loss or theft.**

§483.10(i)(2) Housekeeping and maintenance services necessary to maintain a sanitary, orderly, and comfortable interior;

§483.10(i)(3) Clean bed and bath linens that are in good condition;

§483.10(i)(4) Private closet space in each resident room, as specified in §483.90 (e) (2)(iv);

§483.10(i)(5) Adequate and comfortable lighting levels in all areas;

§483.10(i)(6) Comfortable and safe temperature levels. Facilities initially certified after October 1, 1990 must maintain a temperature range of 71 to 81°F; and

§483.10(i)(7) For the maintenance of comfortable sound levels.

DEFINITIONDS §483.10(i)

"Adequate lighting" means levels of illumination suitable to tasks the resident chooses to perform or the facility staff must perform.

"Comfortable lighting" means lighting that minimizes glare and provides maximum resident control, where feasible, over the intensity, location, and direction of lighting to meet their needs or enhance independent functioning.

"Comfortable and safe temperature levels" means that the ambient temperature should be in a relatively narrow range that minimizes residents' susceptibility to loss of body heat and risk of hypothermia, or hyperthermia, or and is comfortable for the residents.

"Comfortable sound levels" do not interfere with resident's hearing and enhance privacy when privacy is desired and encouraged interaction when social participation is desired. Of particular concern to comfortable sound levels is the resident's control over unwanted noise.

"Environment" refers to any environment in the facility that is frequented by residents, including (but not limited to) the residents' rooms, bathrooms, hallways, dining areas, lobby, outdoor patios, therapy areas and activity areas.

A **"homelike environment"** is one that de-emphasizes the institutional character of the setting, to the extent possible, and allows the resident to use those personal belongings that support a homelike environment. A determination of "homelike" should include the resident's opinion of the living environment.

"Orderly" is defined as an uncluttered physical environment that is neat and well-kept.

"Sanitary" includes, but is not limited to, preventing the spread of disease-causing organisms by keeping resident care equipment clean and properly stored. Resident care equipment includes, but is not limited to, equipment used in the completion of the activities of daily living.

F635
(Rev. 173, Issued: 11-22-17, Effective:11-28-17; Implementation:11-28-17)
§483.20(a) Admission orders

At the time each resident is admitted, the facility must have physician orders for the resident's immediate care.

INTENT §483.20(a)

To ensure each resident receives necessary care and services upon admission.

GUIDANCE §483.20(a)

"Physician orders for immediate care" are those written and/or verbal orders facility staffs need to provide essential care to the resident, consistent with the resident's mental and physical status upon admission to the facility. These orders should, at a minimum, include dietary, medications (if necessary) and routine care to maintain or improve the resident's functional abilities until staff can conduct a comprehensive assessment and develop an interdisciplinary care plan.

F636
(Rev. 173, Issued: 11-22-17, Effective: 11-28-17, Implementation: 11-28-17)
§483.20 Resident Assessment

The facility must conduct initially and periodically a comprehensive, accurate, standardized reproducible assessment of each resident's functional capacity.

§483.20(b) Comprehensive Assessments

§483.20(b)(1) Resident Assessment Instrument. A facility must make a comprehensive assessment of a resident's needs, strengths, goals, life history and preferences, using the resident assessment instrument (RAI) specified by CMS. The assessment must include at least the following:

(i)   Identification and demographic information
(ii)   Customary routine.
(iii)   Cognitive patterns.
(iv)   Communication.
(v)   Vision.
(vi)   Mood and behavior patterns.
(vii)   Psychological well-being.
(viii)   Physical functioning and structural problems.
(ix)   Continence.

(x)   Disease diagnosis and health conditions.

(xi)   Dental and nutritional status.

(xii)   Skin Conditions.

(xiii)   Activity pursuit.

(xiv)   Medications.

(xv)   Special treatments and procedures.

(xvi)   Discharge planning.

(xvii) Documentation of summary information regarding the additional assessment performed on the care areas triggered by the completion of the Minimum Data Set (MDS).

(xviii) Documentation of participation in assessment. The assessment process must include direct observation and communication with the resident, as well as communication with licensed and no licensed direct care staff members on all shifts.

§483.20(b)(2) When required. Subject to the timeframes prescribed in §413.343(b) of this chapter, a facility must conduct a comprehensive assessment of a resident in accordance with the timeframes specified in paragraphs (b)(2)(i) through (iii) of this section. The timeframes prescribed in §413.343(b) of this chapter do not apply to CAHs.

(i)   Within 14 calendar days after admission, excluding readmissions in which there is no significant change in the resident's physical or mental condition. (For purposes of this section, "readmission" means a return to the facility following a temporary absence for hospitalization or therapeutic leave.)

        ***

(ii)   Not less than once every 12 months.

INTENT §483.20(b)(1)-(2)(i) & (iii)

To ensure that the Resident Assessment Instrument (RAI) is used, in accordance with specified format and timeframes, in conducting comprehensive assessments as part of an ongoing process through which the facility identifies each resident's preferences and goals of care, functional and health status, strengths and needs, as well as offering guidance for further assessment once problems have been identified.

DEFINITIONS §483.20(b)(1)-(2)(i) & (iii)

"**Minimum Data Set**": The Minimum Data Set (MDS) is part of the U.S. federally mandated process for clinical assessment of all residents in Medicare or Medicaid-certified nursing homes. It is a core set of screening, clinical and financial status elements, including common definitions and coding categories, which forms the foundation of a comprehensive assessment.

"**Care Area Assessment (CAA) Process**" is a process outlined in Chapter 4 of the MDS manual designed to assist the assessor to systematically interpret the information recorded on the MDS. Once a care area has been triggered, nursing home providers use current, evidence-based clinical resources to conduct as assessment of the potential problem and determine whether or not to care plan for it. The CAA process helps the clinician to focus on key issues identified during the assessment process so that decisions as to whether and how to intervene can be explored with the resident. This process has three components:

- **Care Area Triggers (CATs)** are specific resident responses for one or a combination of MDS elements. The triggers identify residents who have or at risk for developing specific functional problems and require further assessment.
- **Care Area Assessment (CAA)** is the further investigation of triggered areas, to determine if the care area triggers require interventions and care planning.
- **CAA Summary** (Section V of the MDS) provides a location for documentation of the care area(s) that have triggered from the MDS, the decisions made during the CAA process regarding whether or not to proceed to care planning, and the location and date of the CAA documentation.

"**Comprehensive Assessment**" includes the completion of the MDS as well as the CAA process, followed by the development and/or review of the comprehensive care plan. Comprehensive MDS assessments include Admission, Annual, Significant Change in Status Assessment and Significant Correction to Prior Comprehensive Assessment.

"**Resident Assessment Instrument (RAI)**" consists of three basic components: the Minimum Data Set (MDS) version 3.0, the Care Area Assessment (CAA) process and the RAI utilization guidelines. The utilization of these components of the RAI yields information about a resident's functional status, strengths, weaknesses, and preferences, as well as offering guidance on further assessment once problems have been identified.

"Utilization Guidelines" provides instructions for when and how to use the RAI. The Utilization Guidelines are also known as the Long-Term Care Facility Resident Assessment Instrument 3.0 User's Manual.

Remarks

Remarks - As nurse managers you know the importance of the MDS. You know that your documentation must be accurate to reflect the care and services you and your direct care staff are providing for the residents. And you also know the adage that if it is not documented that means the care and services was/were not provided. If you are not quite clear about certain matters or if you have questions that may affect your accuracy in documentation, refer those questions to your directors of nursing or to the MDS Coordinator. One of the areas of confusion in documentation is residents' activities of daily living (ADLs). For example, an evening shift staff may have the tendency to document the level of activity the day shift nurse or nurse aide document, which may be different from the level of activity that happened for the evening shift. Accuracy of documentation is very important.

There is the need for in-services in the area of clinical assessment for nurses, as well as accuracy of documentation for nurse aides. Another care area where clinical intervention may not be provided when they should is resident change in condition. A delay in observing resident change in condition may lead to transfer of the patient to the hospital, if the appropriate intervention was not provided timely. This is one of the clinical areas where regular educational in-services is needed for the nursing staff. The MDS Coordinator should also stay abreast of the changes in the MDS Guidelines, attend seminars as needed, and provide in-services for the clinical team at the facility.

For the nurses, please keep your State Operations Manual handy and refer to it as you must; and for the MDS Coordinator, refer to your MDS Manual as you also must.

F637
(Rev. 173, Issued 11-22-17, Effective: 11-28-17, Implementation: 11-28-17)

§483.20(b)(2)(ii) Within 14 days after the facility determines, or should have determined, that there has been a significant change in the resident's physical or mental condition. (For purpose of this section, a "significant change" means a major decline or improvement in the resident's status that will not normally resolve itself without further intervention by staff or by implementing standard disease-related clinical interventions, that has an impact on more than one area of

the resident's health status, and requires interdisciplinary review or revision of the care plan, or both.)

INTENT §483.20(b)(2)(ii)

To ensure that each resident who experiences a significant change in status is comprehensively assessed using the CMS-specified Assessments Instrument (RAI) process.

DEFINITIONS §483.20(b)(2)(ii)

"Significant Change" is a major decline or improvement in a resident's status that 1) will not normally resolve itself without intervention by staff or by implementing standard disease-related clinical interventions; the decline is not considered "self-limiting" (NOTE: Self-limiting is when the condition will normally resolve itself without further intervention or by staff implementing standard clinical interventions to resolve the condition,): 2) impacts more than one area of the resident's health status; and 3) requires interdisciplinary review and/or revision of the care plan. This does not change the facility's requirement to immediately consult with a resident's physician of changes as required under 42 CFR §483.10(i)(14), F580

"Significant Change in Status Assessment (SCSA)" is a comprehensive assessment that must be completed when the Interdisciplinary Team (IDT) has determined that a resident meets the significant change guidelines for either major improvement or decline.

"Assessment Reference Date (ARD)" is the specific end point for the look-back periods in the Minimum Data Set (MDS) assessment process. This look-back period is also called the observation or assessment period.

Remarks

Remarks – Due to the importance of the concept of "significant change in residents' condition", I recommend that you pay very close attention to the definitions and guidance of this F-tag, including the list of examples of significant changes. In this guidance section CMS is reminding direct care givers and MDS coordinators that if there is only one change, the resident may still benefit from a SCSA if the IDT determines this to be the case, and also if it is initiated in the residents' care plan. The Care Area

Assessment (CAA) must be completed within 14 days after the determination is made that there is change in condition. Also note that according to CMS, a Significant Change MDS is considered timely if the RN Coordinator signs the MDS as complete at section Z0500B & V0200B2 by the 14th calendar day after the determination that a significant change has occurred.

(Refer to the State Operations Manual Appendix PP for the full content of F637 guidance).

Below are the examples that are cited as decline and improvements for significant change as referenced in the guidance section.

A Significant Change in Status, MDS is required when:

- A resident enrolls hospice program; or
- A resident may change hospice providers and remains in the facility; or
- A resident receiving hospice services discontinues those services; or
- A resident experiences a consistent pattern of changes, with either **two or more** areas of decline or **two or more** areas of improvement, from baseline (as indicated by comparison of the resident's current status to the most recent CMS-required MDS).

Examples of Decline include, but not limited to:

- Resident's decision-making ability has changed;
- Presence of a resident mood item not previously reported by the resident or staff and/or an increase in the symptom frequency, e.g., increase in the number of areas where behavioral symptoms are coded as being present and/or the frequency of a symptom increases for items in Section E behavior;
- Changes in frequency or severity of behavioral symptoms of dementia that indicate progression of the disease process since last assessment.
- Any decline in an ADL physical functioning area (at least 1) where a resident is newly coded as Extensive assistance, Total dependence, or Activity did not occur since last assessment and does not reflect normal fluctuations in that individual's functioning;
- Resident's incontinence pattern changes or there was placement of an indwelling catheter;
- Emergence of unplanned weight loss problem (5% change in 30 days or 10% change in 180 days).

- Emergence of a new pressure ulcer at Stage 2 or higher, or a new unstageable pressure ulcer/injury, a new deep tissue injury or worsening of the pressure ulcer status.
- Resident begins to use restraint any type; when it was not used before;
- Emergence of a condition or disease in which a resident is judged to be unstable.

Examples of Improvement include, but not limited to:

- Any improvement in ADL physical functioning area (at least 1) where a resident is newly coded as Independent, Supervision, or Limited assistance since last assessment and does not reflect normal fluctuations in that individual's functioning;
- Decrease in the number of areas where behavioral symptoms are coded as being present and/or the frequency of a symptom decreases;
- Resident's decision making ability improves;
- Resident's incontinence pattern improves;

F641
(Rev. 211: Issued: 02-03-23; Effective: 10-21-22; Implementation: 10-24-22)
§483.20(g) Accuracy of Assessments.
The assessment must accurately reflect the resident's status.

INTENT §483.20(g)

To assure that each resident receives an accurate assessment, reflective of the resident's status at the time of the assessment, by staff qualified to assess relevant care areas and are knowledgeable about the resident's status, needs, strengths, and areas of decline.

GUIDANCE §493.20(g) (this is an abridged form of the guidance; refer to State Operations Manual Appendix PP for the full content of the guidance)

"Accuracy of Assessment" means that the appropriate, qualified health professional correctly document the resident's medical, functional, and psychosocial problems and identify resident strengths to maintain or improve medical status, functional abilities, and psychosocial status using the appropriate Resident Assessment Instrument (RAI) (i.e. comprehensive, quarterly, significant change in status).

F655
(Rev. 173, Issued: 11-22-17; Effective: 11-28-17; Implementation: 11-28-17)
§483.21 Comprehensive Person-Centered Care Planning

§483.21(a) Baseline Care Plans

§482.21(a)(1) The facility must develop and implement a baseline care plan for each resident that includes the instructions needed to provide effective and person-centered care of the resident that meet professional standards of quality care. The baseline care plan must---

(i)	Be developed within 48 hours of a resident's admission.
(ii)	Include the minimum healthcare information necessary to properly care for a resident including, but not limited to—

> A. Initial goals based on admission orders.
> B. Physician orders.
> C. Dietary orders.
> D. Therapy services.
> E. Social services.
> F. PASARR recommendation, if applicable

§483.21(a)(2) The facility may develop a comprehensive care plan in place of the baseline care plan if the comprehensive care plan—

(i)	Is developed within 48 hours of the resident's admission.
(ii)	Meets the requirements set forth in paragraph (b) of this section (excepting paragraph (b)(2)(i)) of this section).

§483.21(a)(3) The facility must provide the resident and their representative with a summary of the baseline care plan that includes but is not limited to:

(i)	The initial goals of the resident.
(ii)	A summary of the resident's medications and dietary instructions.
(iii)	Any services and treatments to be administered by the facility and personnel acting on behalf of the facility.
(iv)	Any updated information based on the details of the comprehensive care plan, as necessary.

INTENT §483.21(a)

Completion and implementation of the baseline care plan within 48 hours of a resident's admission is intended to promote continuity of care and communication among nursing home staff, increase resident safety, and safeguard against adverse events that are most likely to occur right after admission; and to ensure the resident and representative, if applicable, are informed of the initial plan for delivery of care and services by receiving a written summary of the baseline care plan.

GUIDANCE §483.21(a) (This is an abridged form of the guidance; refer to the current State Operations Manual for the full content of the guidance)

Nursing homes are required to develop a baseline care plan within the first 48 hours of admission which provides instructions for the provision of effective and person-centered care to each resident. This means that the baseline care plan should strike a balance between conditions and risks affecting the resident's health and safety, and what is important to him or her, within the limitations of the baseline care plan timeframe.

F656
(Rev. 211; Issued: 02-03-23; Effective: 10-21-22; Implementation: 10-24-22)
§483.21(b) Comprehensive care Plans

§483.21(b)(1) The facility must develop and implement a comprehensive person-centered care plan for each resident, consistent with the resident rights set forth at §483.10(c)(2) and §483.10(c)(3), that includes measurable objectives and timeframes to meet a resident's medical, nursing, and mental and psychosocial needs that are identified in the comprehensive assessment. The comprehensive care plan must describe the following—

    (i)   **The services that are to be furnished to attain or maintain the resident's highest practicable physical, mental, and psychosocial well-being as required under §483.24, §483.25 or §483.40; and**

    (ii)   **Any services that would otherwise be required under §483.24, §483.25 or §483.40 but are not provided due to the resident's exercise of rights under §483.10, including the right to refuse treatment §483.10(c)(6).**

    (iii)   **Any specialized services or specialized rehabilitative services the nursing facility will provide as a result of PASARR recommendations. If a facility disagrees with the findings of the PASARR, it must indicate its rationale in the resident's medical record.**

    (iv)   **In consultation with the resident and the resident's representative(s)—**

        A. The resident's goals for admission and desired outcomes.

B. **The resident's preference and potential for future discharge. Facilities must document whether the resident's desire to return to the community was assessed and any referrals to local contact agencies and/or other appropriate entities, for this purpose.**

C. **Discharge plans in the comprehensive care plan, as appropriate, in accordance with the requirements set forth in paragraph (c) of this section.**

"§483.21(b)(3) The services provided or arranged by the facility; as outlined by the comprehensive care plan, must—

(iii)   **Be culturally-competent and trauma-informed.**

INTENT

Each resident will have a person-centered comprehensive care plan developed and implemented to meet his or her preferences and goals, and address the resident's medical, physical, mental and psychosocial needs.

DEFINITIONS

"Culture" is the conceptual system that structures the way people view the world—it is the particular set of beliefs, norms, and values that influence ideas about the nature of relationships, the way people live their lives, and the way people organize their world. Adopted from Substance Abuse and Mental Health Services Administration. Improving Cultural Competence, Treatment Improvement Protocol (TIP) Series No. 59 HHS Publication No. (SMA) 14-4849. https://store.samhsa.gov/system/files/sma14-4849.pdf.

"Cultural Competency" is a developmental process in which individuals or institutions achieve increasing levels of awareness, knowledge, and skills along a cultural competence continuum. Cultural competence involves valuing diversity, conducting self-assessments, avoiding stereotypes, managing the dynamics of differences, acquiring and institutionalizing cultural knowledge, and adapting to diversity and cultural contexts in communities. US Department of Health and Human Services publication: A Blueprint for Advancing and Sustaining CLAS Policy and Practice at: https://www.thinkculturalhealth.hhs.gov/clas/blueprint.

"Resident's Goal" refers to the resident's desired outcomes and preferences for admission, which guide decision-making during care planning.

"Interventions" are actions, treatments, procedures, or activities designed to meet an objective.

"Measurable" is the ability to be evaluated or quantified.

"Objective" is a statement describing the results to be achieved to meet the resident's goals.

"Person-centered care" means to focus on the resident as the locus of control and support the resident in making their own choices and having control over their daily lives.

"Trauma-informed care" is an approach to delivering care that involves understanding, recognizing and responding to the effects of all types of trauma. SA trauma-informed approach to care delivery recognizes the widespread impact, and signs and symptoms of trauma in residents, and incorporates knowledge about trauma into acre plans, policies, procedures and practices to avoid re-traumatization. Adapted from: SAMHSA's Concept of Trauma and Guidance for a Trauma-Informed Approach, https://store. samhsa.gov/system/files/sma14-4884.pdf

GUIDANCE (this is an abridged form of the guidance; refer to the State Operations Manual for the full content of the guidance)

Through the care planning process, facility staff must work with the resident and his/ her representative, if applicable, to understand and meet the resident's preferences, choices and goals during their stay at the facility. The facility must establish, document and implement the care and services to be provided to each resident to assist in attaining or maintaining his or her highest practicable quality of life. Care planning drives the type of care and services that a resident receives. If care planning is not complete, or is inadequate, the consequences may negatively impact the resident's quality of life, as well as the quality of care and services received.

Facilities are required to develop care plans that describe the resident's medical, nursing, physical, mental and psychosocial needs and preferences and how the facility will assist in meeting these needs and preferences. Care plans must include person-specific, measurable objectives and timeframes in order to evaluate the resident's progress toward his/her goal(s).

Care plans must be person-centered and reflect the resident's goals for admission and desired outcomes.

F657
(Rev. 173; Issued: 11-22-17; Effective: 11-28-17; Implementation: 11-28-17)
§483.21(b) Comprehensive Care Plans
§483.21(b)(2) A comprehensive care plan must be---

(i) Developed within 7 days after completion of the comprehensive assessment.

(ii) Prepared by an interdisciplinary team, that includes but is not limited to—

   A. **The attending physician.**
   B. **A registered nurse with responsibility for the resident.**
   C. **A nurse aide with responsibility for the resident.**
   D. **A member of food and nutrition services staff.**
   E. **To the extent practicable, the participation of the resident and the resident's representative(s). An explanation must be included in a resident's medical record if the participation of the resident and their resident representative is determined not practicable for the development of the resident's care plan.**
   F. **Other appropriate staff or professionals in disciplines as determined by the resident's needs or as requested by the resident.**

(iii) Reviewed and revised by the interdisciplinary team after each assessment, including both the comprehensive and quarterly review assessments.

INTENT of §483.21(b)(2)

To ensure the timelines of each resident's person-centered, comprehensive care plan, and to ensure that the comprehensive care plan is reviewed and revised by an interdisciplinary team composed of individuals who have knowledge of the resident and his/her needs, and that each resident and resident representative, if applicable, is involved in developing the care plan and making decision about his or her care.

DEFINITIONS

"Non-physician practitioner (NPP)" is a nurse practitioner (NP), clinical nurse specialist (CNS) or physician assistant (PA).

GUIDANCE §483.21(b)(2) (this is an abridged form of the guidance; refer to the State Operations Manual Appendix PP for the full content)

Facility staff must develop the comp0rehensive care plan within seven days of the completion of the comprehensive assessment (Admission, Annual or Significant Change in Status) and review and revise the care plan after each assessment. "After each assessment" means after each assessment known as the Resident Assessment Instrument (RAI) or Minimum Data Set (MDS) as required by §483.20, except discharge assessment. For newly admitted residents, the comprehensive care plan must be completed within seven days of the completion of the comprehensive assessment and no more than 21 days after admission.

Remarks

Remarks - Nurse Managers, I am also including Quality of Life and Quality of Care in your section, due to the importance of these two fundamentals of the Federal and State Long Term Care Regulations. Your roles as the managers and clinicians make you and what you do essential to patient outcomes. As direct caregivers, your observations and assessments of the residents, your interaction with the residents, your interaction and communication with the nurse aides, and your interaction and communication with all members of the IDT contribute towards an understanding of the needs of the residents. Meeting those needs is crucial to the provision of Quality of Life and Quality of Care for the residents. Below are the F-Tags for Quality of Life and Quality of Care. Another important concept and approach that you and other members of the team need to embrace is the person-centered care and services to meet the individualized care needs of the residents.

F675
(Rev. 211; Issued: 02-03-23; Effective: 10-21-22; Implementation: 10-24-22)
§483.24 Quality of Life

Quality of Life is a fundamental principle that applies to all care and services provided to facility residents. Each resident must receive and the facility must provide the necessary care and services to attain or maintain the highest practicable physical,

mental, and psychosocial well-being, consistent with the resident's comprehensive assessment and plan of care.

INTENT

The intent of this requirement is to specify the facility's responsibility to create and sustain an environment that humanizes and individualizes each resident's quality of life by:

- Ensuring all staff, across all shifts and departments, understand the principles of quality of life, and honor and support these principles for each resident; and
- Ensuring that the care and services provided are person-centered, and honor and support each resident's preferences, choices, values and beliefs.

DEFINITIONS §483.24

"Person Centered Care" – For the purpose of this subpart, person-centered care means to focus on the resident as the locus of control and support the resident in making their own choices and having control over their daily lives. (Definitions - §483.5)

"Pervasive" For the purpose of this guidance, pervasive means spread through or embedded within every part of something.

"Quality of Life" refers to an individual's sense of well-being, level of satisfaction with life and feeling of self-worth and self-esteem. For nursing home residents, this includes a basic sense of satisfaction with oneself, the environment, the care received, the accomplishments of desired goals, and control over one's life." Adapted from the 1986 Institute of Medicine (IOM) published report "Improving the Quality of Care in Nursing Homes," Located at: https://www.ncbi.nlm.nih.gov/books/NBK217548/#ddd00037

Remarks

Remarks – It is stated in the regulation that Quality of Life is a fundamental principle that applies to all care and services. So it is incumbent on you as nurse managers who are directly involved in the day to day care of the residents to embrace this principle. Negative patient outcomes could sometimes be the result of lack of understanding and lack of application of this important principle.

GUIDANCE §483.24 (This is an abridged form of the guidance; refer to the State Operations Manual for the full content of the guidance)

Noncompliance at F675 identifies outcomes which rise to the level of immediate jeopardy and reflect an environment of pervasive disregard for the quality of life of the facility's residents. This can include the cumulative effect of noncompliance at other regulatory tags on one or more residents. To cite noncompliance at F675, the survey team must have evidence that outcomes at other regulatory tags demonstrate a pervasive disregard for the principles of quality of life.

F676
(Rev. 173; Issued: 11-22-17, Effective: 11-28-17, Implementation: 11-28-17)

§483.24(a) Based on the comprehensive assessment of a resident and consistent with the resident's needs and choices, the facility must provide the necessary care and services to ensure that a resident's abilities in activities of daily living do not diminish unless circumstances of the individual's clinical condition demonstrate that such diminution was unavoidable. This includes the facility ensuring that:

§483.24(a)(1) A resident is given the approach treatment and services to maintain or improve his or her ability to carry out the activities of daily living, including those specified in paragraph (b) of this section....

§483.24(b) Activities of daily living.

The facility must provide care and services in accordance with paragraph (a) for the following activities of daily living:

§483.24(b)(1) Hygiene – bathing, dressing, grooming, and oral care,
§483.24(b)(2) Mobility – transfer and ambulation, including walking,
§483.24(b)(3) Elimination-toileting,
§483.24(b)(4) Dining-eating, including meals and snack,
§483.24(b)(5) Communication, including

> **(i)   Speech,**
> **(ii)   Language,**
> **(iii) Other functional communication systems.**

F677
(Rev. 173, Issued: 11-22-17, Effective: 11-28-17, Implementation: 11-28-17)

§483.24(a)(2) A resident who is unable to carry out activities of daily living receives the necessary services to maintain good nutrition, grooming, and personal and oral hygiene; and

DEFINITIONS

"**Oral care**" refers to the maintenance of a healthy mouth, which includes not only teeth, but the lips, gums, and supporting tissues. This involves not only activities such as brushing of teeth or oral appliances, but also maintenance of oral mucosa.

"**Speech, language or other functional communication systems**" refers to the resident's ability to effectively communicate requests, needs, opinions, and urgent problems; to express emotion, to listen to others and to participate in social conversation whether in speech, writing, gesture, behavior, or a combination of these (e.g. a communication board or electronic augmentative communication device).

"**Assistance with the bathroom**" refers to the resident's ability to use the toilet room (or commode, bedpan, urinal); transfer on/off the toilet, clean themselves, change absorbent pads or briefs, manage ostomy or catheter, and adjust clothes.

"**Transfer**" refers to resident's ability to move between surfaces – to/from: bed, chair, wheelchair, and standing positions, (Excludes to/from bath/toilet.)

GUIDANCE (This is an abridged form of the guidance; refer to the State Operations Manual Appendix PP for the full content of the guidance)

The existence of a clinical diagnosis shall not justify a decline in a resident's ability to perform ADLs unless the resident's clinical picture reflects the normal progression of the disease/ condition has resulted in an unavoidable decline in the resident's ability to perform ADLs. Conditions which may demonstrate an unavoidable decline in the resident's ability to perform ADLs include but are not limited the following:

- The natural progression of a debilitating disease with known functional decline
- The onset of an acute episode causing physical or mental disability while the resident is receiving care to restore or maintain functional abilities; and
- The resident's or his/her representative's decision to refuse care and treatment to restore or maintain functional abilities after efforts by the facility to inform and educate about the benefits/risks of the proposed care and treatment:...."

- Note also that depression is a potential cause of excess disability and, where appropriate, therapeutic interventions should be initiated. Follow up if the resident shows signs/symptoms of depression even if not indicated on his or her MDS.

F684
(Rev. 173, Issued: 11-27-17, Effective: 11-28-17, Implementation: 11-28-17)
§483.25 Quality of care

Quality of care is a fundamental principle that applies to all treatment and care provided to facility residents. Based on the comprehensive assessment of a resident, the facility must ensure that residents receive treatment and care in accordance with professional standards of practice, the comprehensive person-centered care plan, and the residents' choices, including but not limited to the following

INTENT

To ensure facilities identify and provide needed care and services that are resident centered, in accordance with the resident's preferences, goals for care and professional standards of practice that will meet each resident's physical, mental, and psychosocial needs.

DEFINITIONS

"Highest practicable physical, mental, and psychosocial well-being" is defined as the highest possible level of functioning and well-being, limited by the individual's recognized pathology and normal aging process. Highest practicable is determined through the comprehensive resident assessment and by recognizing and competently and thoroughly addressing the physical, mental or psychosocial needs of the individual.

"Hospice Care" means a comprehensive set of services described in Section 1861(dd)(1) of the Act, identified and coordinated by an interdisciplinary group (IDG) to provide for the physical, psychosocial, spiritual, and emotional needs of a terminally ill patient and/or family members, as delineated in a specific patient plan of care. (42 CFR §418.3)

"Palliative care" means patient and family-centered care that optimizes quality of life by anticipating, preventing, and treating suffering. Palliative care throughout the continuum of illness involves addressing physical, intellectual, emotional, social, and spiritual needs and to facilitate patient autonomy, access to information, and choice. (§418.3)

"Terminally ill" means that the individual has a medical prognosis that his or her life expectancy is 6 months or less if the illness runs its normal course. (§418.3)

GUIDANCE (This is an abridged form of the guidance; refer to the State Operations Manual Appendix PP for the full content of the guidance)

NOTE: Although Federal requirements dictate the completion of RAI assessments according to certain time frames, standards of good clinical practice dictate that the clinical assessment process is more fluid and should be ongoing. The lack of ongoing clinical assessment and identification of changes in condition, to meet the resident's needs between required RAI assessments should be addressed at §483.35 Nursing Services, F726 (competency and skills to identify and address a change in condition), and the relevant outcome tag, such as §483.12 Abuse, §483.24 Quality of Life, §483.25 Quality of Care, and/or §483.40 Behavioral Health.....

Nursing homes must place priority on identifying what each resident's highest practicable well-being is in each of the areas of physical, mental and psychosocial health. Each resident's care plan must reflect person-centered care, and include resident choices, preferences, goals, concerns/needs, and describe the services and care that is to be furnished to attain or maintain, or improve the resident's highest practicable physical, mental and psychosocial well-being. ....

F692
(Rev. 173, Issued: 11-22-17, Effective: 11-28-17, Implementation: 11-28-17)
§483.25(g) Assisted nutrition and hydration.

(Includes naso-gastric and gastrostomy tubes, both percutaneous endoscopic gastrostomy and percutaneous endoscopic jejunostomy, and enteral fluids). Based on a resident's comprehensive assessment, the facility must ensure that a resident—

§483.25(g)(1) Maintains acceptable parameters of nutritional status, such as usual body weight or desirable body weight range and electrolyte balance, unless the resident's clinical condition demonstrates that this is not possible or resident preferences indicate otherwise;

§483.25(g)(2) Is offered sufficient fluid intake to maintain proper hydration and health;

§483.25(g)(3) Is offered a therapeutic diet when there is a nutritional problem and the health care provider orders a therapeutic diet.

INTENT §483.25(g)

The intent of this requirement is that the resident maintains, to the extent possible, acceptable parameters of nutritional and hydration status and that the facility:

- Provides nutritional and hydration care and services to each resident, consistent with the resident's comprehensive assessment;
- Recognizes, evaluates, and addresses the needs of every resident, including but not limited to, the resident at risk or already experiencing impaired nutrition and hydration; and
- Provides a therapeutic diet that takes into account the resident's clinical condition, and preferences, when there is a nutritional indication.

DEFINITIONS §483.25(g)

Definitions are provided to clarify clinical terms related to nutritional status.

"Acceptable parameters of nutritional status" refers to factors that reflect that an individual's nutritional status is adequate, relative to his or her overall condition and prognosis, such as weight, food/fluid intake, and pertinent laboratory values.

"Artificial nutrition and hydration" are medical treatments and refers to nutrition that is provided through routes other than the usual oral route, typically by placing a tube directly into the stomach, the intestine or a vein.

"Clinically significant" refers to effects, results, or consequences that materially affect or are likely to affect an individual's physical, mental, or psychosocial well-being either positively by preventing, stabilizing, or improving a condition or reducing a risk, or negatively by exacerbating, causing, or contributing to a symptom, illness or decline in status.

"Dietary supplements" refers to herbal and alternative products that are not regulated by the Food and Drug Administration and their composition is not standardized. Dietary supplements must be labeled as such and must not be represented for use as a conventional food or as the sole item of a meal or the diet.

"**Health Care Provider**" includes a physician, physician assistant, nurse practitioner, or clinical nurse specialist, or a qualified dietitian or other qualified nutrition professional acting within their state scope of practice and to whom the attending physician has delegated the task. For issues related to delegation to dietitians, refer to §483.60(e)(2) F808.

"**Nutritional status**" includes both nutrition and hydration status.

"**Nutritional Supplements**" refers to products that are used to complement a resident's dietary needs (e.g., calorie or nutrient dense drinks, total parenteral products, enteral products, and meal replacement products).

"**Therapeutic diet**" refers to a diet ordered by a physician or other delegated provider that is part of the treatment for a disease or clinical condition, to eliminate, decrease, or increase certain substances in the diet (e.g. sodium or potassium), or to provide mechanically altered food when indicated.

"**Tube feeding**" refers to the delivery of nutrients through a feeding tube directly into the stomach, duodenum, or jejunum. It is also referred to as an enteral feeding.

GUIDANCE §483.25(g) – (This is an abridged form of the guidance; refer to the State Operations Manual Appendix PP for the full content of the guidance)

It is important to maintain adequate nutritional status, to the extent possible, to ensure each resident is able to maintain the highest practicable level of well-being. The early identification of residents with, or at risk for, impaired nutrition or hydration status may allow the interdisciplinary team ton develop and implement interventions to stabilize or improve nutritional status before complications arise. Body weight and laboratory results can often be stabilized or improved with time, but may not be correctable in some individuals. Intake alone is not the only factor that can affect nutritional status. Resident conditions and co-morbidities may prevent improved nutritional or hydration status, despite improved intake.

Examples of other factors that may impact weight and the significance of apparent weight changes include the resident's usual weight through adult life, current medical conditions, diet and supplement orders, recent changes in dietary intake, and edema.

"Suggested parameters for evaluating significance of unplanned and undesired weight loss are:

Interval	Significant Loss	Severe Loss
1 month	5%	Greater than 5%
3 months	7.5%	Greater than 7.5%
6 months	10%	Greater than 10%

The following formula determines percentage of weight loss:

% of body weight loss = (Usual weight – actual weight) / (usual weight) x 100

Weight-Related Interventions: For at risk residents, the care plan should include nutritional interventions to address underlying risks and causes of unplanned weight loss or unplanned weight gain, based on the comprehensive or any subsequent nutritional assessment. The development of these interventions should involve the resident and/or the resident representative to ensure the resident's needs, preferences and goals are accommodated.

F693
(Rev. 173, Issued: 11-22-17, Effective: 11-28-17, Implementation: 11-28-17)
§483.25(g) Assisted nutrition and hydration.

(Includes naso-gastric and gastrostomy tubes, both percutaneous endoscopic gastrostomy and percutaneous endoscopic jejunostomy, and enteral fluids). Based on a resident's comprehensive assessment, the facility must ensure that a resident—

§483.25(g)(4)-(5) Enteral Nutrition

§483.25(g)(4) A resident who has been able to eat enough alone or with assistance is not fed by enteral methods unless the resident's clinical condition demonstrates that enteral feeding was clinically indicated and consented to by the resident; and

§483.25(g)(5) A resident who is fed by enteral means receives the appropriate treatment and services to restore, if possible, oral eating skills and to prevent complications of enteral feeding including but not limited to aspiration pneumonia, diarrhea, vomiting, dehydration, metabolic abnormalities, and nasal-pharyngeal ulcers.

DEFINITIONS §483.25(g)(4)-(5)

"**Bolus feeding**" is the administration of a limited volume of enteral formula over brief periods of time.

"**Continuous feeding**" is the uninterrupted administration of enteral formula over extended periods of time.

"**Enteral feeding**" (also referred to as "tube feeding") is the delivery of nutrients through a feeding tube directly into the stomach, duodenum, or jejunum.

"**Feeding tube**" refers to a medical device used to provide liquid nourishment, fluids, and medications by bypassing oral intake. There are two basic categories, naso-grastric and gastrostomy. The type of feeding tube used must be based on clinical assessment and needs of the resident since there are various kinds of feeding tubes within each category.

"**Gastrostomy tube**" (G-tube") is a tube that is placed directly into the stomach through an abdominal wall incision for administration of food, fluids, and medications. The most common type is a percutaneous endoscopic gastrostomy (PEG) tube.

"**Jejunostomy tube**" (a.k.a "percutaneous endoscopic jejunostomy" (PEJ or J-tube") is a feeding tube placed directly into the small intestine.

"**Naso-gastric tube**" ("NG tube") is a tube that is passed through the nose and down through the nasopharynx and esophagus into the stomach.

"**Transgastric jejunal feeding tube**" (G-J tube") is a feeding tube is placed through the stomach into the jejunum and that has dual ports to access both the stomach and the small intestine.

GUIDANCE §483.25 (This is an abridged form of the guidance; refer to the State Operations Manual for the full content of the guidance)

A decision to use feeding tube has a major impact on a resident and his or her quality of life. It is important that any decision regarding the use of a feeding tube br based on the resident's clinical condition and wishes, as well as applicable federal and state laws and regulations for decision making about life-sustaining treatments.

F725
(Rev. 211; Issued: 02-03-23; Effective: 10-21-22; Implementation: 10-24-22)
§483.35 Nursing Services

The facility must have sufficient nursing staff with the appropriate competencies and skills sets to provide nursing and related services to assure resident safety and attain or maintain the highest practicable physical, mental, and psychosocial well-being of each resident, as determined by resident assessments and individual plans of care and considering the number, acuity and diagnoses of the facility's resident population in accordance with the facility assessment required at §483.70(e).

§483.35(a) Sufficient Staff

§483.35(a)(1) The facility must provide services by sufficient numbers of each of the following types of personnel on a 24-hiur basis to provide nursing care to all residents in accordance with resident care plans:

(i)	**Except when waived under paragraph (e) of this section, licensed nurses; and**
(ii)	**Other nursing personnel, including but not limited to nurse aides.**

§483.35(a)(2) Except when waived under paragraph [(e)] of this section, the facility must designate a licensed nurse to serve as a charge nurse on each tour of duty.

INTENT §483.35(a)(1)-(2)

To assure that there is sufficient qualified nursing staff available at all times to provide nursing and related services to meet the resident the residents' needs safely and in a manner that promotes each resident's rights, physical, mental and psychosocial well-being.

DEFINITIONS §§493.35(a)(1)-(2)

"**Nurse Aide**" as defined in §483.5, is any individual providing nursing or nursing-related services to residents in a facility. This term may also include an individual who provides these services through an agency or under contract with the facility, but is not a licensed health professional, a registered dietitian, or someone who volunteers to provide such services without pay. Nurse aides do not include those individuals who furbish services to residents only as paid feeding assistants as defined in §488.301.

GUIDANCE §483.35(a)(1)-(2) (This is an abridged form of the guidance; refer to the State Operations Manual for the full content of the guidance)

Many factors must be considered when determining whether or not a facility has sufficient staff to care for residents' needs, as identified through the facility assessment, resident assessments, and as described in their plan of care. A staffing deficiency under this requirement may or may not be directly related to an adverse outcome to a resident's care or services. It may also include the potential for physical or psychological harm.

As required under Administration at F838, §483.70(e) an assessment of the resident population is the foundation of the facility assessment and determination of the level of sufficient staff needed. It must include an evaluation of diseases, conditions, physical or cognitive limitations of the resident population's, acuity (the level of severity of residents' illnesses, physical, mentaland and cognitive limitations and conditions) and any other pertinent information about the residents that may affect the services the facility must provide.

F726
(Rev. 173, Issued: 11-22-17, Effective: 11-28-17, Implementation: 11-28-17)
§483.35 Nursing Services

The facility must have sufficient nursing staff with the appropriate competencies and skills sets to provide nursing and related services to assure resident safety and attain or maintain the highest practicable physical, mental, and psychosocial well-being of each resident, as determined by resident assessments and individual plans of care and considering the number, acuity and diagnoses of the facility's resident population in accordance with the facility assessment required at §483.70(e).

§483.35(a)(3) **The facility must ensure that licensed nurses have the specific competencies and skill sets necessary to care for residents' needs, as identified through resident assessments, and described in the plan of care.**

§483.35(a)(4) **Providing care includes but is not limited to assessing, evaluating, planning and implementing resident care plans and responding to resident's needs.**

§483.35(c) **Proficiency of nurse aides.**

The facility must ensure that nurse aides are able to demonstrate competency in skills and techniques necessary to care for residents' needs, as identified through resident assessments, and described in the plan of care.

INTENT §483.35(a)(3)-(4),(c)

To assure that all nursing staff possess the competencies and skill sets necessary to provide nursing and related services to meet the residents' needs safely and in a manner that promotes each resident's rights, physical, mental and psychosocial well-being.

DEFINITIONS §483.35

"**Competency**" is a measurable pattern of knowledge, skills, abilities, behaviors, and other characteristics that as individual needs to perform work roles or occupational functions successfully.

GUIDANCE §483.35(a)(3)-(4),(c) (This is an abridged form of the guidance; refer to State Operations Manual for the full content of the guidance)

All nursing staff must also meet the specific competency requirements as part of their license and certification requirements defined under State law or regulations.

Competency in skills and techniques necessary to care for residents' needs includes but is not limited to competencies in areas such as:

- Resident Rights;
- Person centered care;
- Communication;
- Basic nursing skills;
- Basic restorative services;

- Skin and wound care;
- Medication management;
- Pain management;
- Infection control; Identification of changes in condition;
- Cultural competency.

F727
(Rev. 211; Issued: 02-03-23; Effective: 10-21-22; Implementation: 10-24-22)
§483.35(b) Registered nurse

§483.35(b)(1) Except when waived under paragraph (e) or (f) of this section, the facility must use the services of a registered nurse for at least 8 consecutive hours a day, 7 days a week.

§483.35(b)(2) Except when waived under paragraph (e) or (f) of this section, the facility must designate a registered nurse to serve as the director of nursing on a full time basis.

§483.35(b)(3) The director of nursing may serve as a charge nurse only when the facility has an average daily occupancy of 60 or fewer residents.

DEFINITIONS §483.35(b)

"Full-time" is defined as working 40 or more hours a week.

"Charge Nurse" is a licensed nurse with specific responsibilities designated by the facility that may include staff supervision, emergency coordinator, physician liaison, as well as direct resident care.

PROCEDURE AND GUIDANCE §483.35(b) (this is an abridged form of this guidance; refer to States Operations Manual (SOM) for the full content)

Nurse staffing in nursing homes has a substantial impact on the quality of care and outcomes that residents experience. A registered nurse (RN) is typically responsible for overseeing the care provided to nursing home residents by other staff such as Licensed Practical Nurses (LPN) or Certified Nurse Aides (CNA). The RN is generally responsible for more advanced care activities such as resident assessments, consulting with physicians, and administering intravenous fluids or medications.

Facilities are responsible for ensuring they have an RN providing services at least 8 consecutive hours a day, 7 days a week. However per Facility Assessment requirements at F838, §483.70(e), facilities are expected to identify when they may require the services of an RN for more than 8 hours a day based on the acuity level of the resident population. If it is determined the services 0f an RN are required for more than 8 hours a day, refer to the guidance at F725 related sufficient nurse staffing for further investigation.

F728
(Rev. 173, Issued: 11-22-17, Effective: 11-28-17, Implementation: 11-28-17)
§483.35(d) Requirement for facility hiring and use of nurse aides-
§483.35(d)(1) General rule.

A facility must not use any individual working in the facility as a nurse aide for more than 4 months, on a full-time basis, unless—

(i)   **That individual is competent to provide nursing and nursing related services; and**

(ii)   **(A) That individual has completed a training and competency evaluation program, or a competency evaluation program approved by the State as meeting the requirements of §483.151 through §483.154; or**

 (B) That individual has been deemed or determined competent as provided in §483.150(a) and (b).

§483.35(d)(2) Non-permanent employee.

A facility must not use on a temporary, per diem, leased, or any basis other than a permanent employee any individual who does not meet the requirements in paragraphs (d)(1)(i) and (ii) of this section.

§483.35(d)(3) Minimum Competency

A facility must not use any individual who has worked less than 4 months as a nurse aide in that facility unless the individual-

(i)   **Is a full-time employee in a State-approve training and competency evaluation program;**

(ii)   **Has demonstrated competence through satisfactory participation in a State-approved nurse aide training and competency evaluation program or competency evaluation program; or**

  (iii) **Has been deemed or determined competent as provided in §483.150(a) and (b).**

DEFINITIONS §483.35(d)(1-3)

A "**permanent employee**" is defined as any employee the facility expects to continue working on an ongoing basis.

GUIDANCE §483.35(d)(1-3) (This is an abridged form of the guidance; refer to the State Operations Manual for the full content of the guidance)

If an individual has not successfully completed a nurse aide training or competency evaluation program (NATCEP) program at the time of employment, that individual may only function as a nurse aide if the individual is currently in a NATCEP (**not a competency evaluation program (CEP) alone**) and is a permanent employee in his or her first four months of employment in the facility.

F729
(Rev. 211, Issued: 02-03-23; Effective: 10-21-22; Implementation: 10-24-22)
§483.35(d)(4) Registry verification.

Before allowing an individual to serve as a nurse aide, a facility must receive registry verification that the individual has met competency evaluation requirements unless—

  (i) **The individual is a full-time employee in a training and competency evaluation program approved by the State; or**

  (ii) **The individual can prove that he or she has recently successfully completed a training and competency evaluation program or competency evaluation program approved by the State and has not yet been included in the registry. Facilities must follow up to ensure that such an individual actually becomes registered.**

§483.35(d)(5) Multi-State registry verification.

Before allowing an individual to serve as a nurse aide, a facility must seek information from every State registry established under sections 1819(e)(2)(A) or 1919(e)(2)(A) of the Act that the facility will include information on the individual.

§483.35(d)(6) Required retraining.

If, since an individual's most recent completion of a training and competency evaluation program, there has been a continuous period of 24 consecutive months during none of which the individual provided nursing or nursing-related services for monetary compensation, the individual must complete a new training and competency evaluation program or a new competency evaluation program.

F807
(Rev. 173, Issued: 11-22-17, Effective: 11-28-17, Implementation: 11-28-17)
§483.60(d) Food and drink

Each resident receives and the facility provides—

§483.60(d)(6) Drinks, including water and other liquids consistent with resident needs and preferences and sufficient to maintain resident hydration.

Remarks

Remarks - The guidance for this section emphasizes the fact that nursing homes/skilled nursing facilities must have a program or regimen for distributing drinking water to the residents daily, and nurse managers have that responsibility to stay on top of this routine in your facilities. There are situations when staff leaves water pitcher at the residents' bedside, and depending on the residents physical capabilities, or lack thereof, some residents may need assistance to make sure they consume the water that is left at the bedside. Residents' hydration is essential towards their nutritional and care needs. Of course nurse aides would want to make sure that they follow the residents' plans of care as some residents may have restricted fluid levels based on their diagnosis.

GUIDANCE 483.60(d)(6)

Proper hydration alone is a critical aspect of nutrition among nursing home residents. Individuals who do not receive adequate fluids are more susceptible to urinary tract infections, pneumonia, decubitus ulcers, skin infections, confusion and disorientation.

If a concern is identified regarding maintaining a resident's hydration status or about a resident's fluid restriction, see §483.25(g)(1)-(3), F692, Nutrition/Hydration Status.

F808
(Rev. 173, Issued: 11-22-17, Effective: 11-28-17, Implementation: 11-28-17)
§483.60(e) Therapeutic Diets

§483.60(e)(1) Therapeutic diets must be prescribed by the attending physician.

§483.60(e)(2) The attending physician may delegate to a registered or licensed dietitian the task of prescribing a resident's diet, including a therapeutic diet, to the extent allowed by State law.

INTENT §483.60(e)(1)-(2) – To assure that residents receive and consume foods in the appropriate form and/or the appropriate nutritive content as prescribed by a physician, and/or assessed by the interdisciplinary team to support the resident's treatment, plan of care, in accordance with his her goals and preferences.

GUIDANCE §483.60(e)(1)-(2)

If the resident's attending physician delegates this task he or she must supervise the dietitian and remains responsible for the resident's care even if the task is delegated. The physician would be able to modify a diet order with a subsequent order, if necessary.

F809
(Rev. 173, Issued: 11-22-17, Effective: 11-28-17, Implementation: 11-28-17)
§483.60(f) Frequency of Meals

§483.60(f)(1) Each resident must receive and the facility must provide at least three meals daily, at regular times comparable to normal mealtimes in the community or in accordance with resident needs, preferences, requests, and plan of care.

§483.60(f)(2) There must be no more than 14 hours between a substantial evening meal and breakfast the following day, except when a nourishing snack is served at bedtime, up to 16 hours may elapse between a substantial evening meal and breakfast the following day if a resident group agrees to this meal span.

§483.60(f)(3) Suitable, nourishing alternative meals and snacks must be provided to residents who want to eat at non-traditional times or outside of scheduled meal service times, consistent with the resident plan of care.

DEFINITIONS §483.60(f)(1)-(3)

A "**Nourishing snack**" means items from the basic food groups, either singly or in combination with each other.

"Suitable and nourishing alternative meals and snacks" means that when an alternate meal or snack is provided, it is of similar nutritive value as the meal or snack offered at the normally scheduled time and consistent with the resident plan of care.

Remark

Remarks – The next **F-tag is F810 – Assistive devices**. The importance of this tag is to help staff maintain awareness of the need for the residents to improve or continue to maintain their independence and capability for eating independently as much as possible, so the residents' ADLs do not diminish unintentionally. If the resident requires assistive devices for eating, please provide the assistive device(s) for the resident. Do not substitute the assistive device by asking staff to feed resident. Allow residents to eat using the assistive device(s) by themselves as much as they are able. Of course when residents need help, help must be provided by staff.

F810
(Rev. 173, Issued: 11-22-17, Effective: 11-28-17, Implementation: 11-28-17)
§483.60(g) Assistive devices

The facility must provide special eating equipment and utensils for residents who need them and appropriate assistance to ensure that the resident can use the assistive devices when consuming meals and snacks.

GUIDANCE §483.60(g)

The facility must provide appropriate assistive devices to residents who need them to maintain or improve their ability to eat or drink independently, for example, improving poor grasp by enlarging silverware handles with foam padding, aiding residents with impaired coordination or tremor by installing plate guards, or specialized cups. The facility must also provide the appropriate staff assistance to ensure that these residents can use the assistive devices when eating or drinking.

Remark

Remarks – The next two F-tags speaks to staff competencies. As nurse managers and due to your role as supervisors to some of the direct caregivers, you must also know the requirements about staff competencies. Nursing department staff plays significant roles in promoting and providing the care needs daily for residents to maintain and improve their physical, mental, and psychosocial well-being. The next three F-Tags, F947, F948 and F-949 focus on staff competencies.

F947
(Rev. 211: Issued: 02-03-23; Effective: 10-21-22; Implementation: 10-24-22)
§483.95 Training Requirements
Training topics must include but are not limited to—
§483.95(g) Required in-service training for nurse aides.

In-service training must—

§483.95(g)(1) Be sufficient to ensure the continuing competence of nurse aides, but must be no less than 12 hours per year.

§483.95(g)(2) Include dementia management training and resident abuse prevention training.

§483.95(g)(3) Address areas of weakness as determined in nurse aides' performance reviews and facility assessment at §483.70(e) and may address the special needs of residents as determined by the facility staff.

§483.95(g)(4) For nurse aides providing services to individuals with cognitive impairments, also address the care of the cognitively impaired.

DEFINITIONS

A **"nurse aide"** is defined in §483.5 as any individual providing nursing or nursing-related services to residents in a facility. This term may also include an individual who provides these services through an agency or under a contract with the facility, but is not a licensed health professional, a registered dietitian, or someone who volunteers to provide such services without pay. Nurse aides do not include those individuals who furnish services only as paid feeding assistants as defined in §488.301.

Private duty nurse aides who are not employed or utilized by the facility on a contract, per diem, leased, or other basis, do not come under the nurse training provision and therefore are not required to take the training.

Performance Reviews: the process used to evaluate the performance of staff on a periodic basis, which may be annually.

GUIDANCE §483.95(g) (This is abridged form of the guidance; refer to the State Operations Manual Appendix PP for full content of the guidance.)

All facilities must develop, implement and permanently maintain an in-service training program for nurse aides that is appropriate and effective, as determined by nurse aide performance reviews [see §483.35(d)(7)] and the facility assessment as specified at §483.70(e). Changes to the facility's resident population, the facility's physical environment, staff turnover, and modifications to the facility assessment may necessitate ongoing revisions to the facility's training program.

There are a variety of methods that could be used to provide training. For example, nurse aide training may be facilitated through any combination of in-person instruction, webinars (though, should not be webinars alone) and/or supervised practical training hours and should be reflective of nurse aides' performance reviews in order to address identified weaknesses.

F948
(Rev. 173, Issued: 11-22-17, Effective: 11-28-17, Implementation: 11-28-17)
§483.95(h) Required training of feeding assistants.

A facility must not use any individual working in the facility as a paid feeding assistant unless that individual has successfully completed a State-approved training program for feeding assistants, as specified in §483.160

DEFINITION §483.95(h)

Paid feeding assistant is defined in the regulation at 42 CFR 488.301 as "an individual who meets the requirements specified in §483.60(h)(1) of this chapter and who is paid to feed residents by a facility, or who is used under an arrangement with another agency or organization.

GUIDANCE §483.95(h)

A State-approved training course for paid feeding assistants must include, at a minimum, 8 hours of training in the following:

- Feeding techniques.
- Assistance with feeding and hydration.
- Communication and interpersonal skills.

- Appropriate responses to resident behavior.
- Safety and emergency procedures, including the Heimlich maneuver.
- Infection control.
- Resident rights.
- Recognizing changes in residents that are inconsistent with their normal behavior and the importance of reporting those changes to the supervisory nurse.

A facility must maintain a record of all individuals, used by the facility as feeding assistants, who have successfully completed the training course for paid feeding assistants.

F949
(Rev. 211; Issued: 02-03-23; Effective: 10-21-22; Implementation: 10-24-22)
§483.95 Training Requirements.
Training topics must include but are not limited to----
§483.95(i) Behavioral health.

A facility must provide behavioral health training consistent with the requirements at §483.40 and as determined by the facility assessment at §483.70(e).

GUIDANCE §483.95(i) (This is an abridged form of this guidance; refer to the State Operations Manual Appendix PP for the full content of the guidance)

All facilities must develop, implement, and maintain an effective training program for all staff, which includes, at minimum, training on behavioral health care and services (consistent with §483.40) that is appropriate and effective, as determined by staff need and the facility assessment (as specified at §483.70(e)). For the purposes of this training requirement, staff includes all facility staff, (direct and indirect care functions), contracted staff, and volunteers (training topics as appropriate to role).

Changes to the facility's resident population, staff turnover, the facility's physical environment, and modifications to the facility assessment may require ongoing revisions to the facility's training program.

Remarks

Remark – there is no case study for nurse managers to complete here. I included and addressed nurse managers' responsibilities and nurse aides/nursing assistants' duties in the case studies of the other disciplines and in the director of nursing section in the workbook.

The final chapter is for Quality Assurance and Performance Improvement in the nursing home. This topic should encapsulate all that the staffs do and their involvement in care and services for the residents, whether the staffs are direct care staff and indirect staff – all staff!!

Chapter 13

QUALITY ASSURANCE PERFORMANCE IMPROVEMENT

For All Departments & Disciplines

Below are the F-tags for Quality Assessment and Performance Improvement (QAPI). Administrators, directors of nursing, QAPI directors/coordinators, and all department heads in the facility are members of the QAPI Committee. The administrators and QAPI directors/managers must reinforce to all staff that they have a role to play in the facility's QAPI program. Let staff know that they are indirect members of the committee, because their participation in the committee is essential. They could and should bring important issues that may affect the quality of care and services that may affect the residents' care and facility operation to their department heads who are committee members. Furthermore, nurse aides, and other levels of staff need to be included in the QAPI Committee. Also for department heads, as part of your data collection process you will need to ask questions of and collect data from your staff for the totality, accuracy and completeness of your data..

QAPI F-tags - for all disciplines and departments.

F865
(Rev. 211; Issued: 02-03-23; Effective: 10-21-22; Implementation: 10-24-22)
§483.75(a) Quality assurance and performance improvement (QAPI) program.

Each LTC facility, including a facility that is part of a multiunit chain, must develop, implement, and maintain an effective, comprehensive, data-driven QAPI program that focuses on indicators of the outcomes of care and quality of life. The facility must:

§483.75(a)(1) Maintain documentation and demonstrate evidence of its ongoing QAPI program that meets the requirements of this section. This may include but is not limited to systems and reports demonstrating systematic identification, reporting,

investigation, analysis, and prevention of adverse events; and documentation demonstrating the development, implementation, and evaluation of corrective actions or performance improvement activities;

§483.75(a)(2) Present its QAPI plan to the State Survey Agency no later than 1 year after the promulgation of this regulation;

§483.75(a)(3) Present its QAPI plan to a State Survey Agency or Federal surveyor at each annual recertification survey and upon request during any other survey and to CMS upon request; and

§483.75(a)(4) Present documentation and evidence of its ongoing QAPI program's implementation and the facility's compliance with requirements to a State Survey Agency, Federal surveyor or CMS upon request.

§483.75(b) Program design and scope.

A facility must design its QAPI program to be ongoing, comprehensive, and to address the full range of care and services provided by the facility. It must:

§483.75(b)(1) Address all systems of care and management practices;

§483.75(b)(2) Include clinical care, quality of life, and resident choice;

§483.75(b)(3) Utilize the best available evidence to define and measure indicators of quality and facility goals that reflect processes of care and facility operations that have been shown to be predictive of desired outcomes for residents of aa SNF or NF.

§483.75(b)(4) Reflect the complexities, unique care, and services that the facility provides.

§483.75(f) Governance and leadership

The governing body and/or executive leadership (or organized group or individual who assumes full legal authority and responsibility for operation of the facility) is responsible and accountable for ensuring that:

§483.75(f)(1) An ongoing QAPI program is defined, implemented, and maintained and addresses identified priorities.

§483.75(f)(2) The QAPI program is sustained during transitions in leadership and staffing;

§483.75(f)(3) the QAPI program is adequately resourced, including ensuring staff time, equipment, and technical training as needed;

§483.75(f)(4) The QAPI program identifies and prioritizes problems and opportunities that reflect organizational process, functions, and services provided to residents based on performance indicator data, and resident and staff input, and other information.

§483.75(f)(5) Corrective actions address gaps in systems, and are evaluated for effectiveness; and

§483.75(f)(6) Clear expectations are set around safety, quality, rights, choice, and respect.

§483.75(h) Disclosure of Information.

A State or the Secretary may not require disclosure of the records of such committee except in so far as such disclosure is related to the compliance of such committee with the requirements of this section.

§483.75(i) Sanctions.

Good faith attempts by the committee to identify and correct quality deficiencies will not be used as a basis for sanctions.

INTENT

These requirements are intended to ensure that long term care facilities (including multi-unit chains) implement a comprehensive QAPI program which addresses all the care and unique services a facility provides.

DEFINITIONS

"**Governing body**" refers to individuals such as facility owner(s), Chief Executive Officer(s), or other individuals who are legally responsible to establish and implement policies regarding the management and operations of the facility.

"**Indicators**" are measurement(s) of performance related to a particular care area or service.

"**Quality Assurance and Performance Improvement (QAPI)**" is the coordinated application of two mutually-reinforcing aspects of a quality management system: Quality Assurance (QA) and Performance Improvement (PI). QAPI takes a systematic, interdisciplinary, comprehensive, and data-driven approach to maintaining and improving safety and quality in nursing homes while involving residents and families in practical and creative problem solving.

"**Quality Assurance (QA)**" is the specification of standards for quality of service and outcomes, and systems throughout the organization for assuring that care is maintained at acceptable levels in relation to those standards. QA is on-going, both anticipatory and retrospective in its efforts to identify how the organization is performing, including where and why facility performance is at risk or failed to meet standards.

"**Performance Improvement (PI)**" (also called Quality Improvement – QI) is the continuous study and improvement of processes with the intent to improve services or outcomes, and prevent or decrease the likelihood of problems, by identifying areas of opportunity and testing new approaches to fix underlying causes of persistent/systemic problems or barriers to improvement. PI in nursing homes aims to improve processes involved in health care delivery and resident quality of life. PI can make good quality even better.

GUIDANCE

QAPI is a type of quality management program which takes a systematic, interdisciplinary, comprehensive, and data-driven approach to maintaining and improving safety and quality. An interdisciplinary approach encompasses all managerial, and clinical, services, which includes care and services provided by outside (contracted or arranged) providers and suppliers.

The purpose of a QAPI program is to ensure continuous evaluation of facility systems with the objectives of:

- Ensuring care delivery systems function consistently, accurately, and incorporate current and evidence-based practice standards where available;
- Preventing deviation from care processes, to the extent possible;

- Identifying issues and concerns with facility systems, as well as identifying opportunities for improvement; and
- Developing and implementing plans to correct and/or improve identified areas.

QAPI Plan

A QAPI plan is the written plan containing the process that will guide the nursing home's efforts in assuring care and services maintained at acceptable levels of performance and continually improved. The plan describes how the facility will conduct its required QAPI and QAA committee functions. The facility is required to develop a QAPI plan and present its plan to federal and state surveyors at each annual recertification survey and upon request during any other survey, and to CMS upon request.

The QAPI plan should describe the scope of the QAA committee's responsibilities and activities, and the process addressing how the committee will conduct the activities necessary to identify and correct quality deficiencies. Each nursing home, including facilities which are a part of a multi-chain organization, should tailor its QAPI plan to reflect the specific units, programs, departments, and unique population it serves, as identified in its facility assessment.

The QAPI plan should describe how the facility will ensure care and services delivered meet accepted standards of quality, identify problems and opportunities for improvement, and ensure progress toward correction or improvement is achieved and sustained.

The QAPI plan should describe the process for identifying and correcting quality deficiencies. Key components of the process include:

- Tracking and measuring performance;
- Establishing goals and thresholds for performance measurement;
- Identifying and prioritizing quality deficiencies;
- Systematically analyzing underlying causes of systemic quality deficiencies;
- Developing and implementing corrective action or performance improvement activities; and
- Monitoring or evaluating the effectiveness of corrective action/performance improvement activities, and revising as needed.

(For additional content information for F865 refer to State Operations Manual (SOM))

F866
(Rev. 211; Issued: 02-03-23; Effective: 10-21-22; Implementation: 10-24-22)
Note: Regulatory requirements §483.75(c) and §483.75(c)(1)-(4) have been relocated to F867

F867
(Rev. 211; Issued: 02-03-23; Effective: 10-21-22; Implementation: 10-24-22)
§483.75(c) Program feedback, data systems and monitoring,

A facility must establish and implement written policies and procedures for feedback, data collections systems, and monitoring, including adverse event monitoring. The policies aand procedures must include, at a minimum, the following:

§483.75(c)(1) Facility maintenance of effective systems to obtain and use of feedback and input from direct care staff, other staff, residents, and resident representatives, including how such information will be used to identify problems that are high risk, high volume, or problem-prone, and opportunities for improvement.

§483.75(c)(2) Facility maintenance of effective systems to identify, collect, and use data and information from all departments, including but not limited to the facility assessment required at §483.70(e) and including how such information will be used to develop and monitor performance indicators.

§483.75(c)(3) Facility development, monitoring, and evaluation of performance indicators, including the methodology and frequency for such development, monitoring, and evaluation.

§483.75(c)(4) Facility adverse event monitoring, including the methods by which the facility will systematically identify, report, track, investigate, analyze and use data and information relating to adverse events in the facility, including how the facility will use the data to develop activities to prevent adverse events.

§483.75(d) Program systematic analysis and systemic action.

§483.75(d)(1) The facility must take actions aimed at performance improvement and, after implementing those actions, measure its success, and track performance to ensure that improvements are realized and sustained.

§483.75(d)(2) The facility will develop and implement policies addressing:

    (i)   How they will use a systematic approach to determine underlying causes of problems impacting larger systems;

    (ii)   How they will develop corrective actions that will be designed to effect change at the systems level to prevent quality of care, quality of life, or safety problems; and

    (iii)   How the facility will monitor the effectiveness of its performance improvement activities to ensure that improvements are sustained.

§483.75(e) Program activities.

§483.75(e)(1) The facility must set priorities for its performance improvement activities that focus on high-risk, high-volume, or problem-prone areas; consider the incidence, prevalence, and severity of problems in those areas; and affect health outcomes, resident safety, resident autonomy, resident choice, and quality of care.

§483.75(e)(2) Performance improvement activities must track medical errors and adverse resident events, analyze their causes, and implement preventive actions and mechanisms that include feedback and learning throughout the facility.

§483.75(e)(3) As part of their performance improvement activities, the facility must conduct distinct performance improvement activities, the facility must conduct distinct performance improvement projects. The number and frequency of improvement projects conducted by the facility must reflect the scope and complexity of the facility's services and available resources, as reflected in the facility assessment required at §483.70(e). Improvement projects must include at least annually a project that focuses on high risk or problem-prone areas identified through the data collection and analysis described in paragraph (c) and (d) of this section.

§483.75(g) Quality assessment and assurance.

§483.75(g)(2) The quality assessment and assurance committee reports to the facility's governing body, or designated person functioning as a governing body regarding its activities, including implementation of the QAPI program required under paragraphs (a) through (e) of this section. The committee must:

    (ii)   Develop and implement appropriate plans of action to correct identified quality deficiencies;

    (iii)   Regularly review and analyze data, including data collected under the

QAPI program and data resulting from drug regimen reviews, and act on available data to make improvements.

INTENT

These provisions are intended to ensure facilities obtain feedback, use data, and take action to conduct structured, systematic investigations and analysis of underlying causes or contributing factors of problems affecting facility-wide processes that impact quality of care, quality of life, and resident safety.

DEFINITIONS

"Adverse Event" is defined in §483.5 as an untoward, undesirable, and usually unanticipated event that causes death or serious injury, or the risk thereof.

"Corrective Action": A written and implemented plan of action for correcting or improving performance in response to an identified quality deficiency. Use of the term corrective action in this guidance is not synonymous with a Plan of Correction (formal response to cited deficiencies). This is also separate from the written QAPI plan.

"High-risk areas": Refers to care or service areas associated with significant risk to the health or safety of residents. Errors in these care areas have the potential to cause ad verse events resulting in pain, suffering, and/or death. Examples include tracheostomy care; pressure injury prevention; administration of high-risk medications such as anticoagulants, insulin, and opioids.

"High-volume areas": Refers to care or service areas performed frequently or affecting a large population, thus increasing the scope of the problem, e.g., transcription of orders; medication administration; laboratory testing.

"Incidence": is a measure of the number of new cases of a characteristic that develop in a [population in a specified time period. National Institute of Mental Health (NIMH) (https://www.nimh.nih.gov/health/statistics/what-is-prevalence.shtml. Accessed

"Indicator" measurement of performance related to a particular care area or service delivered. Used to evaluate the success of a particular activity in achieving goals or thresholds.

"**Medical Error**": is a deviation from the process of care, which may or may not cause harm to the resident.

"**Near Miss**": is a serious error or mishap that has the potential to cause an adverse event that fails to do so because of chance or because it is intercepted. It is also called a potential adverse event.

"**Prevalence**": is the proportion of a population who have a specific characteristic in a given time period. NIMH (https://www.nimh.nih.gov/health/statistics/what-is-prevalence.shtml, accessed 12/21/2020).

"**Problem-prone areas**": Refers to care or service areas that have historically had repeated problems, e.g., call bell response times; staff turnover; lost laundry.

"**Quality Assurance and Performance Improvement (QAPI)**": Nursing home QAPI is the coordinated application of two mutually-reinforcing aspects of a quality management system" Quality Assurance (QA) and Performance Improvement (PI). QAPI takes a systematic, interdisciplinary, comprehensive, and data-driven approach to maintaining and improving safety and quality in nursing homes while involving residents and families, and all nursing home caregivers in practical and creative problem solving.

- **Quality Assurance (QA)**: QA is the specification of standards for quality of care, service and outcomes, and systems throughout the facility for assuring that care is maintained at acceptable levels in relation to those standards. QA is on-going and both anticipatory and retrospective in its efforts to identify how the organization is performing, including where and why facility performance is at risk or has failed to meet standards.
- **Performance Improvement PI)**: PI (also called Quality Improvement – QI) is the continuous study and improvement of processes with the intent to improve services or outcomes, and prevent or decrease the likelihood of problems, by identifying opportunities for improvement, and testing new approaches to fix underlying causes of persistent/systemic problems or barriers to improvement. PI in nursing homes aims to improve facility process involved in care delivery and enhanced resident quality of life. PI can make good quality even better.

"**Quality Deficiency (or Opportunity for Improvement)**": A deviation in performance resulting in an actual or potential undesirable outcome, or an opportunity for improvement. A quality deficiency is anything the facility considers to be in need of further investigation and correction or improvement. Examples include problems such as medical errors and accidents, as well as improvement opportunities such as responses to questionnaires showing decreased satisfaction. This term is not necessarily synonymous with a noncompliance deficiency cited by surveyors, but may include issues related to deficiencies cited on annual or compliant surveys.

"Systematic": describes a step by step process that is structured, so that it can be replicated.

"Systemic": embedded within, and affecting a system or process.

GUIDANCE (This is abridged form of the guidance; refer to the State Operations Manual Appendix PP for the full content of the guidance)

As required in §483.75(a) (F865), the facility must develop and implement systems that ensure the care and services it delivers meet acceptable standards of quality in accordance with recognized standards of practice. This is accomplished, in part, by identifying, collecting, analyzing and monitoring data which reflects the functions of each department and outcomes to residents.

Feedback

Feedback is one of many data sources which provide valuable information the facility must incorporate into an effective QAPI program. Each facility must establish and implement written policies and procedures for feedback.

Feedback must be obtained from direct care staff, other staff, residents and resident representatives as well as other sources, and be used to identify problems that are high-risk, high-volume, and/or problem-prone, as well as opportunities for improvement. Feedback fro residents is necessary to understand what quality concerns are important to them, their perspectives, values and priorities, as well as impact of the facility's daily routines on their physical, mental, and psychosocial well-being. Staff can also provide valuable input into understanding care and service delivery processes.

A facility should choose the best mechanism for feedback to support their QAPI program. Examples of mechanisms for obtaining resident and staff feedback may include, but are not limited to:

- Satisfaction surveys and questionnaires;

- Routine meetings, e.g. care plan meetings, resident council, safety team, town hall; and
- Suggestion or comment boxes

Effective feedback systems in a QAPI program also include methods for providing feedback to direct care staff, residents and representatives. This may involve including these individuals in problem solving, various meetings or providing updates and communicating facility system changes.

Data Collection Systems and Monitoring

In order to ensure care and services are carried out consistently, accurately, timely and according to recognized standards of quality, the facility must collect and monitor data reflecting its performance, including adverse events.

Facility policies and procedures must address how data will be identified, and the frequency and methodology for collecting and using data from all departments. The facility determines what data it will collect to represent its care areas considered to be associates with high-risk, high-volume, and/or problem-prone issues.

Data collection can be done using several methods, such as audit tools (purchased or developed by the facility), direct observation, interview, or testing. Sources for data may include the Minimum Data Set (MDS) and Quality Measures, electronic and paper medical records, survey results, incident reports, complaints, suggestions and staffing data. CMS expects the data collection methodology to be consistent, reproducible and accurate to produce data that are valid and reliable, and support all departments and the facility assessment (§483.70(e).

It is not necessary to collect all data at the same frequency. The facility may develop a schedule for routine data collection

I am ending the workbook with these few words, which I hope you will find useful.

A Demanding yet Rewarding Career

Long term care is in fact a rewarding career, as we manage all the day to day challenges that come with the profession and career. Providing the care and services for the residents although demanding at times depending on the situation, helps provide that sense that you are doing something good that moves the residents forward in their recovery and/or in their level of comfort. Sometimes you as the staff become the family for some of the residents who may not have visits from families or who may not even have families. So keep your chin up when you feel down sometimes.

In the midst of the concerns, issues and complaints from residents, from families, from advocates, from government agencies both federal and state agencies, just bear in mind that these are not criticisms, but are comments and concerns to make us do better, and improve on our systems for better outcomes. The voluminous regulations sometimes get us overwhelmed and stressed, but you will get through and become familiar with the F-tags. I know it is not easy, but you have the courage and determination as long term care professionals and workers to work through the challenges. You have what it takes to continue to make a positive difference in the lives of your residents. You sacrifice your time sometimes, when you are asked to work beyond your regular work hours, although you may have committed that time to be with your families You are appreciated for being a difference maker and a team player.

There have been some trying times in the industry, and staffing has been and continues to be one of the trying times. Not enough staff affects quality, and this continues to test the resiliency of the industry. You show that you are devoted and committed employees, devoted to the love for your job, the residents, and for your fellow employees - members of the team.

This is to thank you for all that you continue to do, and to appreciate you for your hard work and commitment as I know, speaking from experience, that this is not an easy career path, but a beautiful and rewarding career path.. So thank you, thank you, and thank you!!!

References

State Operations Manual Appendix PP – Guidance to Surveyors for Long Term Care Facilities – Rev. 211, 02-03-23

U.S. Department of Health & Human Services, Office of Inspector General: Nursing Homes Featured Report Last Updated: 10-03-2023

U.S. Department of Health & Human Services, Office of Inspector General: Data Brief: Trends in Nursing Home Deficiencies (A-09-18-02010)

Advancing Excellence in America's Nursing Homes – Commonwealth Fund

Design for Nursing Home Compare Five-Star Quality Rating System, Technical Users' Guide April 2019 . Centers For Medicare & Medicaid Services

Design for Care Compare Nursing Home Five-Star Quality Rating System: Technical Users' Guide September 2023.

Centers For Medicare & Medicaid Services

Printed in the United States
by Baker & Taylor Publisher Services